THE
BOY
BETWEEN

THE BOY BETWEEN

A Mother and Son's Journey From a World Gone Grey

AMANDA PROWSE
JOSIAH HARTLEY

Little
a

Published by Little A, Seattle

www.apub.com

Amazon, the Amazon logo, and Little A are trademarks of Amazon.com, Inc.,
or its affiliates.

ISBN-13: 9781542022286
ISBN-10: 1542022282

Cover design by James Jones

Printed in the United States of America

My dedication is for all those who are living with depression. For all those who are thinking or have thought that suicide might be the best option. I am proof that there is a life to be lived after depression and a life to be lived with depression – though it might not always feel like it. Don't give up. Talk it through, write it down, run, dance, read, paint, sleep, play sport, do yoga, sit in a chair, walk in a park! Do whatever you need to and wait it out until the demon is off your back and the darkness passes. Take a breath. Take a moment. As I say in the book, things can and often do get better. Don't delete yourself.

DON'T DO THAT.

Don't wipe out what just might be a fantastic future. The world is big. The possibilities infinite. Know that the world is better with you in it. It's a shit hard struggle – probably the hardest you will ever face, but you can do it.

I did it.
I do it.
I know you can too.

Josh

I would like to dedicate this book to all those who care for and all those who love someone suffering with depression or mental illness. Yours is not always the easier ride, but a different one and arguably the one with less support. Know that when you cry tears of frustration, when you howl at the moon for want of direction, when the questions are many but the answers few and when your body aches at the end of another hard day spent with muscles coiled in tension, you are not alone. We are one of many even though loving those who suffer in this way can feel like the loneliest job in the world. We are one of many even though it often feels like no one can possibly understand how we live, and we are one of many even when it feels like no one cares.

YOU ARE NOT ALONE!

I think, for us, this phrase by Pablo Casals is pertinent: 'To the whole world you might be just one person, but to one person you might just be the whole world.' For those we love and care for this can often be the truth. What an incredible responsibility! But, oh my, what an incredible privilege . . .

Amanda Xx

We wrote this book based on our memories of the events in question. Some events have been compressed and some dialogue has been recreated from memory. We have aimed to be truthful in all we've told but accept that our memory is fallible.

CONTENTS

PROLOGUE

Josh

The decision to end my life was one that came easily. There was not, as you might imagine, some great wrangling with the consequences of something so final. None at all. By the time I came to the conclusion that to slip away from this existence was probably the best thing for me, I had lost the ability to think deeply about anything or anyone. I was beyond reason, with my reality skewed. I wasn't sad. I was numb. This state felt interminable. I was exhausted, and the thought of having to spend the rest of my days in this endless blank circle of desperation was one I was not prepared to contemplate. What was the point?

I woke that day in the mental fog I had grown accustomed to. All thoughts were slow and slurred, making rational thinking improbable. It must have been daytime as the sun rather unsuccessfully shone through my perpetually drawn blinds. A few weeks prior, looking out at the blue sky was almost a treat, something to break up the monotony of the day, but I was past that now. Time had lost all meaning: I could have been in that room anywhere between five days to three weeks, sleeping up to eighteen hours a day and spending the other six in a trance-like haze, staring up at the ceiling. My bed was an island; it happened to be in a medium-sized UK city, but in terms of loneliness and isolation it might as well have been in the South Pacific. I occasionally left my island to get water, food or use the loo, but recently even thirst had failed me. The pull of that bed was like trying to escape a black hole. I felt beyond the event horizon and even the greatest invitation of all time would not have tempted me away from that six-foot by four-foot space that was my world.

I was unaware of my surroundings but looking back they were fairly putrid. The studio flat in which my illness had fully taken grip could have been the student dream – a large space for one person, with brand-new appliances and all the creature comforts, laying the foundation for an excellent year. But dirty clothes and old takeaway containers were stuck to the wooden floor. My sheets hadn't been washed for months and I had no timescale to work with for when I'd last showered. It didn't matter though; nothing did. The very colour of the world had turned down until only greyscale remained.

Day by day over an unknown period of time my emotions were chipped away piece by piece, subtly enough for me not to notice. I was an empty husk, devoid of emotion. I wasn't sad anymore; I felt nothing. Being sad would have been an improvement; the ability to feel anything had been gone for quite some time.

I opened the package containing the tablets. The smell of sulphur hit me. They were a solution and therefore something definitive, a marker in a life that had become rootless.

I often think about that boy sitting on the end of the bed with the tablets in his palm. A boy living in the space between darkness and light. I think of how his story nearly ended on that day. I think about his family telling tales of a life that became overwhelming and was now no more than a footnote in their history. I was that boy and it was not my last day, but I came close.

INTRODUCTION

Amanda

It is hard to write with honesty about depression, suicide and all the unpalatable truths that come with both, hard to find the positives and the hope, because it is a dark topic and one that we would rather not talk about, but we are going to try. Josh and I would like to tell the story of what happened when mental illness came to live in our ordinary house with us, an ordinary family. I thought mental illness – frightening, hard to fathom, and even harder to accept – was something that happened to other people. Turns out we are other people. And here we are.

The Boy Between is the account of Josh's depression to the point where he not only considered, but also planned when and how he would end his life – and very nearly succeeded. This is the first time either Josh or I have spoken publicly about the demon that he carries on his back. It has been the hardest thing that we as a family have ever been through, mainly because, as parents, Simeon and I felt woefully ignorant of how to deal with the situation, and partly because mental illness does not always have the neat, predictable, hopeful conclusion that we humans take such comfort from. It's almost as if we can cope with something because we know that the situation won't be forever – but what if it is? Indeed, words of solace are often wrapped in this theme: 'Time is a great healer' and 'Time heals all wounds' and even 'This too shall pass . . .' But with our son's depression there came a moment when we had to accept that maybe none of the above applied. This thought is a devastating one for us and for our son: that he may always be vulnerable and the 'okayish' days of just about coping might actually be as good as it gets. The idea does not get any easier.

This is a book I would have liked to have read at the lowest points on our journey, something I could have reached for when the world felt like a very lonely place and I truthfully questioned everything I held dear, even my own judgement. I often think about all of us who go to bed at night with the knot of worry in our stomachs over our children and I imagine these knots are fashioned from invisible thread that weaves us all together, and that thought brings me comfort because we are stronger together and life is a little better, easier, if we talk about it. In the dead of night, I still doubt all that I usually take for granted – the very pillars on which my life is propped – my parenting style, my people skills, my career choice and even my marriage. Am I the worst mother in the world? Has our other son, Ben, been affected by his brother's illness in ways I do not yet understand? Did I do something to make Josh feel this way? How much more of my mental absence can my husband take? And what might happen to us, as a couple, when our every waking moment is hijacked by Josh's depression that sits like a boulder in the middle of every conversation, just waiting to trip us up? I ask whether I am selfish to write novels, cloistered away in my own little world while things have seemingly spiralled out of control. Did I take my eye off the ball? How can we live as a family like this, how do we function? And crucially, why? Why is it our youngest son ended up in this position without my seeing it coming?

We are, I write with no small measure of pride, one of those families who talk openly around the dining table, where there is no subject that is off limits. The kind of parents who go on holiday with our boys, Josh and Ben, and who make a habit of knowing

4

their friends, partners and their routines; I thought I had it covered. If you had asked, I would have said confidently, even a little smugly, that I knew my kids better than anyone, knew what was going on with them. Turns out I didn't, not at all. And that's a very hard thing for me to accept.

A book like this would, I think, have helped me twofold: first, to know that I was not alone – that other families are also stumbling blindly through this terrible thing; and second, to glean insights from someone suffering, because all I wanted to know was how to help Josh best. I wanted someone to tell me what they had done and how it made things better.

Josh's illness has sledgehammered all that we took for granted, hijacking every thought or enjoyable activity with a deep-seated worry of what our world might look like if and when he were to take his life. It's often all I can think about.

It is relentless.

It is exhausting.

In writing everything down we have had to relive the monstrous events, things we had hoped to forget, and I have again had to face up to the fact that my son wanted to cease living. Recounting certain aspects has certainly been harrowing and yet, bizarrely, what I have learned about his state of mind at the moment of his possible demise is where I take the most comfort.

I cannot adequately explain the hours I have spent in utter despair, awash with self-recrimination, trying to imagine the anguish Josh must have felt at that moment when, all alone, suicide felt like the best option. I have imagined him in a number of guises, but always weeping, desolate and lonely, his adult self juxtaposed with the toddler who used to look at me with big eyes and arms raised at a time when physical comfort and a biscuit could cure just about everything. And the idea that I was not with him in that moment: that he was alone . . . It's the very worst thing for any loving parent to picture and feels a lot like failure.

Josh's words, however, about that actual day have given me a fantastic and welcome insight, dispelling the myth for me and taking away some of the heightened emotion, and I take much comfort from it. Far from feeling the desperate sadness I had envisaged, he told me that if he felt anything at all it was relief; this feeling above all else managed to pierce the armour of numbness in which he was cloaked. It reminded me on a much smaller scale of what it felt like, only an hour after having dropped off a crying Josh at nursery, to receive the call and hear that he was, 'Completely fine now! Playing with Lego and not upset at all! Don't worry a jot . . .'

I remember back then, as a single mum, some eight years before I met Simeon, being able to go about my working day with the knot removed from my gut and awash with relief, able to concentrate on the job in hand, unburdened and, yes, happy. This was the same, but the relief, unburdening and happiness were of course much, much greater.

One of the unexpected privileges of being a writer is that people contact me to share their own stories, many of them heartfelt experiences that often feel a lot like the unburdening of a secret that has been buttoned up in their minds for too long. Lots of these stories have been about loved ones who have taken their own lives. And it is often a staggeringly similar picture that emerges. One man told me about the woman he loved who cooked a final meal of her favourite food and ate it alone, leaving his kitchen in a wonderful state of clutter, and how he now pictured her savouring each mouthful and raising a glass with a smile on her face. This imagining brought him immense comfort. Another detailed how their son went for a glorious hike, whistling as he returned to plant a kiss on his mother's cheek. *She* took great comfort from the fact that he had chosen to bestow upon her his last kiss ever. To her it seemed fitting as she had given him his very first.

There are other suicide stories trustingly shared in confidence, but all spoke of either uplift in the mood and countenance of those who had chosen to take leave of this world or at the very least a calm resignation. I would not attempt anything so crass as to suggest that I begin to understand what these individuals or their loved ones have been through. I don't. Of course I don't. But I will say that I personally took a great deal of comfort from the fact that when the worst thing was about to happen, Josh was calm.

Calm.

And this is a tough one because I will fight until my last breath to keep him with me, to keep him alive. A world without Josh in it is one I simply cannot conceive of, and yet this thought sits like the smallest of paper cuts on the tip of my finger, a constant sharp reminder that happiness and peace are the things I have always wanted for Josh. But at what cost?

My beautiful, perfectly imperfect son sat with suicide pills in the palm of his hand and prepared to leave our lives, to disappear from the face of the earth.

He was nineteen years old.

In writing this I have learned more than I ever thought possible about the inner workings of Josh's mind and his thought processes and I'm in complete admiration of his raw honesty and strength – not only in his ability to articulate the most painful of events, but I also understand a little more about the battle he fights every single day. No wonder he is so tired. I have also learned a lot through his stories and recollections about my own style of parenting, some of it very hard to hear. Yet no matter how hard, it has been necessary, especially if we stand any chance of changing the outcome for our son. Our communication is now more open, more honest and a bit like ripping off a Band Aid that is stuck fast: I wish we had done it quickly and immediately a long, long time ago.

I believe the fact that he is still alive is down to two things: a few simple acts that bought precious time, and a whole lot of luck.

This memoir is written by me, Amanda, Josh's ill-equipped mum doing her very best (and often failing) to say and do the right thing – trying, with her husband by her side, to keep her son alive, working towards his happiness, and by my son, Josiah (Josh), who could, for so long, only see life through the fog of depression and wanted nothing more than for the interminable pain of nothingness to end.

Ours are two distinct voices that speak openly from the heart, charting our very different perspectives on Josh's rollercoaster of a life. I should probably tell you now that this unwanted guest is still in our house, but for now, today at least, it is locked in the attic, held at bay. I should probably also tell you that there is no glorious air-punching moment when I detail Josh's arrival at a place called happiness, or where Simeon and I get to sit back, glass in hand, and reminisce about the bad times.

Josh's depression has become my master too, and it rules me with fear. In quieter moments I hear it rattling the chains and kicking on the door behind which it is locked. My fear has subsided a little but is still present. I am still afraid of doing or saying the wrong thing – fearful that 'the wrong thing' might end up being the straw that breaks his back, the action or phrase that makes him want to take his life. It's like living on a knife-edge with a chasm either side, plus the knife is on fire, I am barefoot, bullets are raining down, I can't breathe, there's an angry dragon circling overhead and no one can hear me call for help . . .

It's a hard thing to write and an even harder thing to say out loud that my son, my beautiful, beloved child who is now a man, suffers with a mental illness that means, some of the time at least, he would prefer not to exist.

Even looking at the words on the page they seem grotesque to me.

He would prefer not to exist . . .

How is this even in his thoughts, and how did it come to the point when he tried to take his life?

He is and always will be the love of my life. It's been harrowing, energy-sapping, spirit-breaking, exhausting; the list of negative adjectives is a long one. But that doesn't mean I would change anything about being Josh's mum. Nothing.

He is my greatest joy and has been since the moment he was first placed in my arms all squash-nosed and tomato-faced. On that day when he was brand new, I wished for him many things but never, ever in a million years did I imagine that the thing I would pray for more than any other was that my beautiful boy didn't kill himself.

But here we are; this is real life and unlike my novels where I get to craft the most ingenious and pleasing situations in which my characters exist, this is not quite how things seem to be turning out. Of course, we are not at the end just yet, there is still time, but right now?

I think the most honest thing to say is that life is . . . unpredictable.

The trouble is, there isn't a map, instruction manual or guidebook. I wish there were. I want someone to tell me how to mend him! To tell me what to do. I want to find that magic tablet that will make it all better. But instead I have to feel my way in the dark and I stumble, often. The truth is there isn't much that life can throw at you that is harder than watching your child suffer. It feels like the cruellest blow. Life with Josh has been a rollercoaster – but one where over the last few years the highs have got lower and the lows lower still. I have repeated to myself, often in the dead of night, in the lonely, dark hours, as I cry in my husband's arms with bedclothes rucked around me and my hair stuck to my face, when thoughts are loudest and sleep evades, that no matter how hard it is for me, for *us* as a family, it is a damn sight harder for Josh.

Not that this is easy to forget – on certain days his face is a haunted picture that drifts from room to room, but those are the bad days and the ones on which I try not to dwell. There are some rare days when he laughs, laughs loudly! And it is the sweetest music in my ears. It is relief, joy and most important it is the sound of hope. And those bursts of hope are the driftwood to which I cling.

Yes, it's hard. And in a phrase that will resonate with all parents, in fact with all those who have loved: Josh's pain is my pain. His joy is my joy and if he wants to jump from the face of the earth in search of peace eternal, then the one thing I know for sure is that he will take my heart and spirit with him. And what would that leave? No more than the husk of me, an aching void of emptiness at my loss.

I am, I confess, preoccupied with how to keep Josh from doing the unthinkable and taking his own life. We are slowly, cautiously, starting to come out the other side, still trying to piece together what happened, how we got there and where we go from here.

When I look back at the last six years, it feels a bit like we were taken up high into the sky by a whirling tornado, which hit with such force we didn't have time to take a breath or make a plan. It turned and spun without respite. It was punishing, exhausting and all we could do was cling on, holding tightly to those closest and hoping that when we landed, intact if we were lucky, we might vaguely recognise the landscape among which we wandered.

This is where we are at, we have landed *almost* intact and we are wandering, dazed and, yes, a little confused, surveying the damage, trying to figure out what *can* be salvaged and actually not mourning all that we have lost, just thankful, beyond thankful, to be back on solid ground with time to breathe. I am filled with happy appreciation of every day on the planet with Josh on it, knowing that while he is still here, there is time.

My name is Amanda, but you can call me Mandy. I am the mum of the boy between, the boy who struggled to see just how brilliant life can be and this is my story.

Chapter One

Amanda

'The day I met the love of my life: my baby boy'

'If I had a flower for every time I thought of you . . .
I could walk through my garden forever.'

Alfred Tennyson

I spend a lot of time thinking back to the days when I was a single mum, trying to figure out what I could and should have done differently that might have meant a different outcome for Josh. There is one particular day that sticks in my mind. I drove across The Downs, a green, wide-open space that graces the city of Bristol. It was early morning and we were on our way to the nursery. Clutching his book bag in his small hand, Josh sat in the passenger seat wearing his little grey shorts and socks that stopped below the knee, summer sandals and a sweatshirt bearing the crest of his fancy school, the fees for which kept me awake most nights. We chatted as we always did, covering topics as varied as the merits of Nutella versus honey and which was his favourite *Bug's Life* character and why. I asked him quite casually what he wanted to be when he grew up. He stared out of the window a little nonplussed and so I threw in some suggestions, hoping, I must now confess with more than a little shame, that one of these seeds might germinate. Paving the way, I thought, for the glorious life that awaited him.

'You could be a doctor? Or an artist, a musician?'

He stayed silent for a while, transfixed by life rumbling by on the blue-sky day as we tootled along, until eventually he turned to me and said, 'I think when I grow up, I'd like to cut the grass on The Downs.'

I laughed, loudly.

'Really, Joshy? You can be anything you want to be. You will have this brilliant life! And you can be anything at all. A playwright or an astronaut exploring space! Think about it, wouldn't you like to climb a mountain or be a surgeon or play music?'

He shook his head and spoke wistfully yet adamantly. 'No, Mum. I think I'd like to cut the grass on The Downs.'

'Why? Why do you want to do that, darling?' I was yet to meet a three-year-old who didn't have wild flights of fancy about their grown-up life. That wonderful time when dreams are not quashed by practicality and the thought of being a lion tamer who also works in a cake shop or a ship's captain who is also a famous drummer in a rock band feels possible. And why not? I admit I was interested, a little perplexed and, again I write with no small dollop of embarrassment, somewhat disappointed by his rather mundane answer. I can now see that this was because I was living Josh's future in my head. And that future looked glorious. I saw him tall, accomplished and running at life with his arms wide, ready to grab armfuls of all that was on offer and really *live*.

Josh returned his gaze to the window and the tanned, laughing faces of the men riding the tractor-style mowers with trailers attached.

'Because they look happy, Mum.'

I thought it was cute and interesting and it was only when I looked at him and he stared back at me with an expression of such sadness that I wanted to weep, realising in that moment that he was striving for something far more elusive than a career in space exploration. *Happiness.*

'Yes, they do, Joshy,' I had to admit. 'They look really happy.'

My brilliant boy had figured out at this tender age something that it took me decades to grasp: that happiness is the goal. That's it: happiness! If you have that then everything else kind of falls into place and nothing else really matters. And it was in this noble pursuit that I was determined to help him.

I didn't know what motherhood would be like before I became a mum – who does? I mean, I had an idea and had, I thought, learned from watching others, my own mother included, but it is a thing that is almost impossible to imagine. I think it's a bit like the difference between *reading* about diving into a swimming pool and actually *doing* it. Sure you know what to expect, can look at pictures or read about technique, safety and even how others have experienced it, but that glorious feeling as your body is immersed in water, as your skin shivers, your heart pounds and your hair floats above you . . . that otherworldly experience where some senses are muted and others heightened, where sounds echo, light is filtered, and if you hover beneath the surface it feels like you have entered another realm entirely – *that* you can only *feel*.

Motherhood, I think, is like that.

Nature is a clever old thing and I know I speak for many when I say that as soon as my son was born – in that very moment – it was almost impossible to imagine a life without him. It was, as they say, love at first sight, or if not love then certainly a bond of devotion that felt a lot like it. And with that love came a passion, a need to protect and nurture my child at all costs. 'Easy-going Mandy' discovered a new side to her character: for the first time ever I knew that I would die trying to stop any harm coming to this child of mine. Even *thoughts* of harm were enough to set my heart racing and my gut tensing in readiness to pounce.

In my more flippant moments when pregnant, in those wonderful hours of daydream with my baby safe and snug in my womb, when everything felt possible and I had no idea how this new human would hijack my every waking thought and how every decision I would ever make would have him at the heart of it, I think if *pressed* I might have guessed that life with my baby would be very similar to a Gap advert. One where I walked calmly in warm tones of oatmeal through a park with my beautiful son alongside me. We would be clad in matching denim, of course, and he might be wearing a natty striped scarf around his neck. I imagined we'd stop to feed the odd duck and I might push him on a swing, laughing as I flicked my shiny hair, relishing having got back into my skinny jeans so quickly and with the sun shining on a blue-sky winter's day. Then we'd come home, probably to something healthy and delicious I'd put in the oven earlier, and I'd bathe the little darling before popping him under a Cath Kidston duvet, where he would sleep for a full twelve hours after a bedtime story. We would then wake smiling and repeat . . . He would grow up happy and beautiful and successful and he'd love me a lot and life would be great.

If only . . .

The babyhood thing was tough, and if I think of it in terms of train stations I can only recall being stuck on the tracks in a go-slow carriage between Exhausted Town and What Happened To My Lifeville. And as for my Gap advert fantasy – it might have been possible if Gap ever decided to tout grubby tunics with baby sick on the shoulder and stretched leggings worn by a model who hasn't washed her hair for a month, sporting the haggard look of the undead due to lack of sleep. The kind of model who cries in the bath because her hormones are in overdrive, frothing and seeping from every orifice, and who, due to a particularly strenuous pregnancy and childbirth, had lost the ability to laugh, cough, hiccup and fart without wetting herself. I thought *everything* would be easier, confident that I just needed to follow the rules. I mean, how hard could it be? I knew the basics: give birth, keep him safe and warm, feed him well, love him enough, be the best example, listen to him, give him self-belief and the freedom to fly, but always, always with a safety net beneath him in case he should fall . . .

I didn't realise he would fall often and his wings would break and that trying to get him to open his eyes, let alone fly, would be the hardest thing of all.

I had many dreams for my newborn boy, but can now, hand on heart, say that I couldn't care less about a job, a title, a vocation or an allocated grade on a shitty exam paper. All I wish is that he finds peace of mind. Even 'happy' often feels like too much to ask for. I could never have imagined that the thing that would keep me awake on many a night was trying to figure out how to keep Josh here. Often during strenuous bouts of tears, people tell me to stick with it and that '*things will get easier* . . .' Well, my baby is now twenty-three and I'm a still a-waitin'!

I can joke.

I do that a lot: laugh or make light of the things that cut my very soul. Because what's the alternative?

Chapter Two

Josh

'I am The Boy Between'

'Every man has his secret sorrows which the world knows not; and often times we call a man cold when he is only sad.'

Henry Wadsworth Longfellow

My name is Josiah. You can call me Josh. I'm twenty-three and I am the boy who, some of the time at least, would prefer not to exist.

It's odd to be telling you – whoever happens to be reading this book about my innermost thoughts – things I have done my best to keep to myself for a long, long time.

It feels like a big deal.

It is a big deal.

I'm nervous, but I know that if I don't talk about it I become part of the problem. Secrecy, stigma, taboo, shame and judgement are enablers of this horrible illness when what we actually need is to expose how common this issue really is and confirm to those suffering that they are not alone.

I hope one day that people will be able to chat in the street or across the water cooler and say, 'I am depressed. I have depression', in the same way we do a cold or the flu. And with the reminder that unlike the flu, you can't catch depression.

I hope my story in some small way will help with this.

I find it surprising – or maybe interesting would be more accurate – how my view on what it's like to exist on this planet seems to be at odds with just about everyone else I encounter. It's not a conscious thing; it's just how it has always been for me. And it's a view I never questioned until I had to, until it turned into something more than a view and became a state of mind. A damaging state of mind.

I don't judge anyone for their differing view and don't expect them to judge me. I just can't imagine being them or living their life – it's the same when I meet people who are chirpy, filled with sunshine, have the conviction of faith or are simply overflowing with hope and optimism, confident that it all turns out all right in the end. They are to me an enigma.

But I'm not morose, just thoughtful. Not introverted, more cautious.

And while others express such joy at simply 'being' I stare at them and wonder if it's just me who finds the whole process of living so very exhausting. And I question how they can avoid or deny the one truth: that none of us gets out of here alive.

To clarify, I'm not a sad person. There are rarely tears. I sometimes think it might be easier if there were, a release if you like. But don't misunderstand me – I don't wake each day with the burden of sadness. In recent times I've often felt joy, lots of it, but if joy is the grass in the garden of my life, you don't have to dig very deep to discover that it's sitting on a solid bedrock of utter despair.

It's a frightening thing, living this way. It's like building your home on a fault line, knowing there is a strong possibility that at some undetermined time, probably when you least expect it, you and everything that makes up your world, all the things you hold dear, might tumble into a gaping void. And so no matter how fine things might seem, even on the brightest of days, this foul possibility sits at the back of your mind. Yes: a bedrock of despair. And it is this despair that has in recent times wrapped around me and threatened to overwhelm me. A despair to which I nearly succumbed.

Depression crept up on me, robbing me of myself, and by the time I fully realised what was happening it was too late; I was in its grip.

Its grip is a powerful one, holding me fast, rendering me both blind and mute. If I believed in such things, I think this comes very close to my definition of hell.

For a long, long time I could see life only through the fog of mental illness, and in truth I wanted nothing more than for the interminable pain of nothingness to end.

It's funny, isn't it, that it's super common to have depression; we hear it every day. Everyone from truck drivers to movie stars, shelf-stackers to chefs – no one is immune and yet one of its dirtiest tricks is that it makes you feel like you are the only one who has ever suffered in this way. And not only are you the only one but, having been muted by the condition that holds you fast, it is almost impossible to tell anyone how you feel – even if you could adequately describe it.

At least that was what it felt like for me.

It is isolating, torturous and monstrously unfair that it can, for people like me, take what should be the best years of our lives. And it robs others of countless opportunities, holding them prisoner. I am thankful that the dialogue about depression is finally opening up. We *are* getting better at discussing mental health – some

18

of the bigger recent campaigns are making a difference, notably those by CALM (Campaign Against Living Miserably) with their 'Grow a Pair' campaign saying plainly that if your mate's struggling, start listening. 'Because sometimes the bravest thing you can do for someone is set everything else aside, including your judgement – and just listen.'[1]

There is also the ITV campaign for mental wellness, which promotes the idea that Britain needs to 'Get Talking' in order to bring families closer together. It states the uncomfortable fact that 'anxiety and depression in children has risen by 48 per cent since 2004. But talking and listening can build mental wellness, so we're encouraging you to tune back into the story in your living room.' 'Britain Get Talking' is supported by YoungMinds and Mind.[2]

And Mind itself, who campaign for better mental health and who are partners in 'Time To Change', which asks us all to 'Rethink Mental Illness, England's most ambitious campaign to end the stigma and discrimination faced by people who experience mental health problems.'[3]

And finally Mental Health America's 'Mental Health Month', which has been running for over seventy years. Their outlook is a refreshing one: 'Much of our work is guided by the Before Stage 4 (B4Stage4) philosophy – that mental health conditions should be treated long before they reach the most critical points in the disease process. When we think about diseases like cancer or heart disease, we don't wait years to treat them. We start before Stage 4 – we begin with prevention, identify symptoms, and develop a plan of action to reverse and hopefully stop the progression of the disease. So why don't we do the same for individuals who are dealing with potentially serious mental illness?'[4]

These are just some of the campaigns that are making a difference, but there is still a long, long way to go before the depression and suicide narrative is greeted without prejudice, without embarrassment and without judgement. And I say that both as someone who has suffered and someone who has judged others. I think people are still learning, adjusting to this new world where suicide is on the rise and still the biggest single killer of men under forty-five in the UK.[5]

I'm still learning and know I will learn a lot by talking to you. You, the stranger I am trusting with my thoughts. I guess in recent times the most valuable thing I have learned is that the smallest thing can lead to a whole heap of hope, and in that moment it can feel a lot like happiness. And when in the grip of depression, where time has no meaning, any moment of relief, any second of hope that gives you a chance to reset, to change the narrative, can mean more than you think. It can be the difference between deciding to go and deciding to stay. I have also learned that I'm stronger than I thought. That sometimes it can feel like the end of the road but it isn't – proof being I am still here.

I AM STILL HERE.

I've learned that it's okay to change direction – and that something that happens in a period of your life doesn't have to, and should not, define the *rest* of your life. At least that is what I am hoping. It's a nice relief to realise that I have a whole lot of living left to do. And I guess most importantly, I now know I wasn't alone even though I felt it. I know this because the people who were there for me then are still here for me now. Looking back, I can now see that this sense of isolation was part of my depression. A nasty trick.

I have also learned not to look too far ahead, as that is where the unknown lurks and that can be a scary thought.

So here we are.

I didn't give up, didn't delete myself, but I came very close.

I know what it feels like to stand on the edge of the abyss and not give a shit about anything other than ending the silent nothingness that feels eternal. I know what it feels like to stand in that

20

place and feel the dark hand of depression gently pushing on your back – encouraging you to do it.

And ironically, I know that in that moment the prospect of escape, of peace, was the one thing that, in as long as I could remember, made me feel the first stirrings of happiness.

I remember saying this aloud for the first time and the look of horror on Mum's face was blatant. I see her fear and have tried to explain that this is not her story.

Not her battle.

It's mine.

Chapter Three

Amanda

'Happy is the goal'

'A mother is the truest friend we have, when trials, heavy and sudden, fall upon us; when adversity takes the place of prosperity; when friends who rejoice with us in our sunshine, desert us when troubles thicken around us, still will she cling to us, and endeavor by her kind precepts and counsels to dissipate the clouds of darkness, and cause peace to return to our hearts.'

Washington Irving

I was never one of those little girls who dreamed of becoming a mother, didn't really have dolls, well, I didn't need them. My mum tells stories of living in our cramped house when my baby brothers would wake up in the night to be fed or changed, and I would jump out of bed and make my way barefoot across the landing in my Ladybird bri-nylon nightie to my parents' room with a weary sigh – I would then sit and hold the little one or chat to Mum while she fed him, as if it was partly my responsibility too. And she would then have to settle us all back to sleep.

An often-shared family story is me appearing at the foot of their bed holding my eight-month-old brother and announcing, 'He needs his bum changing. He's a bloody nightmare!'

I was three.

Can you *imagine*?

A three-year-old carrying a baby around in the middle of the night! This of course was in a time before health and safety had been discovered, a world where dummies (pacifiers) were dipped in whisky to ease a teething baby, where 'baby rice' was put into feeding bottles to ensure a full tum and where mums were told to put babies on their stomachs for sleep. A time when my three brothers and I travelled long journeys, taking it in turns to lie on the parcel shelf of my dad's roomy Ford, and there was a rota as to who could sit in the front on my mum's lap (not so roomy) for a cuddle as we tootled endlessly along, wishing there were more motorways. I am indeed a child of the 1970s and it's a wonder any of us survived.

I think this total immersion in the world of babyhood was probably enough to put me off. I remember at quite a young age sitting in class as my teacher asked us in turn what we wanted to be when we grew up. Someone wanted to be an actress, someone else a footballer, and when it came to me I answered quite simply that I wanted to write books – a lofty ambition in my run-down state school where truancy and indifference were high and ambition, among staff and pupils alike, was low. I remember the look of derision cast in my direction by my teacher – who was sharp, spiky and even her smile was no more than the pressing of thin lips together over her tiny yellow teeth – as if to say, *You? Write a book? Ha!*

And I can still hear the ripple of laughter spreading around the room when one girl announced when she grew up she wanted to be a mum; I can picture her expression of surprise, as if to say doesn't *everyone* want to do that?

Judging by that reaction, I'd say apparently not, Michelle!

So I guess I was more than a little influenced by my own mum, who popped out babies like the rest of us shell peas. At one point she had three children under the age of five. Even writing that gives me a mild panic attack and makes my remaining fallopian tube knot itself. Three under five? What were my parents thinking? I mean, I know we didn't have central heating, but sweet mother of Betsy, there must have been other ways to keep warm.

The funny thing is that despite the noise and clutter, it was the very best time for us all. The very best: magical even. Far from finding it daunting or overwhelming, my dad, fresh out of his teens, worked tirelessly and selflessly, trying to work his way up the corporate ladder by day, shovelling tarmac for the boom in road building at night, and fixing his Ford Corsair on the driveway at weekends, doing anything and everything to keep his family afloat and give us the kind of life he and my mum dreamed of. My mum, equally young, turned our small three-bedroomed, orange-bricked terraced house in Collier Row, Romford, into a haven. I can picture it now with the floors covered in toys, and meals often eaten in a tent made of sheets under the table, as the twin-tub washing machine juddered around the tiny kitchen and her beloved Motown provided the background music to the chaos. I can see her dancing in her denim high-waisted flares with her long, dark, shiny hair about her shoulders and a cigarette held aloft between two fingers, singing along to The Supremes' 'Reflections'. We were loved and cherished and I knew the way I felt about my mum and dad was something wonderful, but I wanted something different – I was bookish and not remotely interested in boys: yuck! Or babies: even yuckier!

Turns out it was a good job, as having been born with a congenital defect to my pelvis and after a dozen gruelling surgeries

24

throughout my young life – it meant the chances of me giving birth were slim. In our house, my physical deformity wasn't a topic of particular interest or even a point of discussion; like the fact that money was scarce and space even scarcer or that my mum and dad fell into bed each night exhausted from parenting and working, it was just how it was. And following the example set by my mum and dad, I took my dodgy pelvis in my (rather wobbly) stride and got on with life. I had after all been raised with the phrase 'Your normal is your normal', and this still rings true for me today.

I do remember a growing concern as a teenager was being able to walk 'normally', wanting nothing more than to be free of my rather awkward gait that one physiotherapist remarked upon to my mother while I was very much in earshot: 'Goodness me, she walks like a pregnant duck!' Stunned, I can't quite remember my mum's response, but I'm pretty sure it ended in 'off!'. I hoped the operations might help relieve me of my waddle. What didn't distress me at that point were the rather rushed phrases and awkward coughs around the fact that I would be highly unlikely to carry a baby to full term. I remember looking at the consultant, who had a somewhat dismissive air, and my mum and dad, who could only see me as the little bookworm I was, and the whole idea of motherhood felt so very alien and so far away that there felt little point in giving it any thought. I was more interested in how I could sneak my mum's copy of *Lace* for a secret read with the aid of a torch under the duvet after lights out than the fact that I might never have a child. The whole subject felt like a thing belonging to a grown-up world that was as remote as it was unimaginable.

Funny also how I treasure this life, this brilliant life, all of it: every bite, every sip, every giggle, every deep breath, every glorious scent, every moment by the ocean, every gaze up into the sky, every interaction with those I love who I know I will lose, every wrinkle, every ache, every sleep-deprived night; and my wish, my *greatest* wish is to show Joshy just how wonderful this life can be. But I mustn't rush ahead . . .

With most of the ambition beaten out of me by my rather crappy educational experience, I left school with no lofty ideas of going into any of the professions and worked hard at a variety of unfulfilling, poorly paid jobs to pay the rent and put food on the table. I papered over the cracks both metaphorically and physically, sticking a poster (David Bowie as Ziggy in case you were wondering) over the patches of mould in my rented room. And I plastered on a smile and three coats of sticky strawberry-scented lip gloss before heading off to work where I spent many minutes in a week dodging the wandering hands of my superiors and trying to 'jest' my way through unwanted suggestions and intimidating remarks that the older me would respond to very differently. I was, like most of us, on the hamster wheel of life, clocking up the hours, taking the wage and covering my bills, just. I drank cheap plonk at the weekends and danced till the early hours in the clubs of London, where my glossed lips were only marginally stickier than the booze-slopped floors on which I bopped, and a bit like my mum I did it in flares and with long hair about my shoulders, but without the cigarette. I would then ride the night bus home, dreaming of a day and a life when I might travel and wake without setting an alarm.

It was when I hit my twenties that the idea of *not* becoming a mum began to bloom into a deeper concern and I started to picture a life where I would be the best auntie in the world to my brothers' future kids, but likely never have my own, and that was okay. Simon, Paul, Nicky and I have always been close, and I knew they would welcome me being a part of their children's lives. I figured that I could find contentment and fulfil my parenting itch through my, as yet unborn, nieces and nephews. I found though that as time marched on the acceptance of my probable childless state turned into something a lot closer to sadness, but a sadness I nevertheless made peace with. I had been raised with the thought 'no one gets all the gifts!' and so babies were, I assumed, one gift, albeit one very big gift, that I would just have to do without.

I was twenty-eight when, newly married, I fell pregnant. Not the miracle you might imagine: getting pregnant was not a problem, it was staying pregnant that was tricky. With each month that passed, I watched incredulously, cautiously, as my stomach grew – and in direct correlation my trepidation rose, fully expecting this pregnancy to end in miscarriage. (I have suffered many, both before and after this pregnancy.) But this baby, much to my utter delight and surprise, I carried to full term.

I didn't *dislike* being pregnant exactly, but neither was I a bump-cradling, info-gathering fanatic, relishing my fatness and eagerly perusing expert books whilst throwing baby showers and planning placenta smoothie quaffing parties. I was somewhere in the middle: happy to be pregnant, inevitably a little afraid, working doubly hard to pay the rent, but with a firm belief that everything would somehow work out how it was meant to. After all, millions of women all over the world since the beginning of humanity had had babies, how hard could it be?

That makes me laugh.

I was so naive.

It was a snowy January when despite the odds Josh hurtled into my world like a meteorite, smashing down my emotional barriers and leaving my life plan in smithereens. And quite frankly, it was a shock! Now, I know I'd had nine months to get used to the idea, but I don't think I fully believed I was going to be given a baby at the end of the episode but, blow me down, that's exactly what happened.

It was somewhat of a miracle when my little boy climbed into the world. I use the word climbed in the most literal sense. Born by caesarean section, he almost reached out his arms and lifted up his head, hastening his own exit from my body and into the big wide world. The Aussie medic who had delivered him raised him up and said, 'I think he's in a hurry, keen to explore!'

And I, along with the whole medical team, laughed.

We laughed in relief because Josh had been safely delivered, we laughed at his antics, and I laughed because I had cheated the system. I was not supposed to become a mum but there he was, my boy: the biggest gift of all and he was mine. I felt afraid; it was surreal that this little human was my responsibility – *me*, the girl my parents said couldn't have a guinea pig because I likely wouldn't take care of it. Now, twenty years had passed since my guinea pig request had been turned down but I was beginning to worry they might have been right. With my confidence low I wasn't sure I did know how to take care of a guinea pig, let alone a baby! I didn't have the foggiest idea what I was supposed to do. But I think this is how we all feel in that moment when you realise this is what you have always longed for and yet you might actually not have the skills to do it properly.

As an exhausted, aching new mum, whose bones felt a little too soft, skin a little pulled and with boobs that felt like they were weighted, I was, it's fair to say, more than a little overwhelmed by the whole experience of giving birth. I was also at the time hanging on to the tailfin of a short-lived marriage that was nose-diving fast, and I wished for no more than sleep and a hot bath. Holding the newly hatched Josh in my arms, I tentatively asked the midwife, 'When will he nod off, do you think?', knowing that when he dozed that was *my* chance to follow suit. I couldn't possibly sleep and leave him awake; I didn't want to miss his first look around at the planet on which he had newly arrived. Plus, I figured he might have questions.

'Oh, any minute now!' she chortled. 'He's been through a lot too, a big day for him. He'll be very tired.'

Tell me about it, Nurse Pamela . . .

Reassured, I sat back against the pillows on the creaky bed with my son swaddled and resting on my raised legs, looking at me, blinking. He was, of course, the most beautiful thing I had ever seen, a tiny creature of such intrigue and wonder, with a little button nose and big blue eyes, framed by envy-inducing lashes. His mouth was a perfect cupid's bow and he sat with his small fists curled under his chin, cherub-like in the pose. I was smitten, a little afraid, but mainly smitten. I knew beyond a doubt that there would never be anything in my life nearly half as good as watching this brand-new human.

'Happy Birthday, little man . . .' I cooed. 'I love you and I'm so pleased to meet you. I'm Mandy, I'm your mum and this is your first day ever . . . You are going to do so many wonderful things . . . so many wonderful things . . .'

I soon ran out of chat and banter when six hours, yes, *six hours* later, he decided to take a nap.

Josh has never ever done what was expected of him.

I think I knew then that this kid was going to carve his own path. And quite frankly the prospect thrilled and terrified me in equal measure.

I looked at him and I wished for him all good things: health, happiness and, I must admit, success. My life was hard and at that moment in time, success to me looked like a great career, a happy home and all the wonderful things to fill it with. I am laughing a different kind of laugh now, one that preludes tears, when I think that I wished for my son material things. Oh, how my wishes have altered over the years.

We named him Josiah after my beloved grandad and this was almost instantly shortened to Josh.

The marriage I referred to did *indeed* hit the ground, and having crawled from the wreckage I became a single mum when Josh was a young toddler. I worked all the hours God sent, sometimes working three or four jobs, cleaning offices and waitressing among other things, following my parents' example that hard work was the way to achieve just about anything and determined to be the best example to him that I could be. With my ex-husband living at the other end of the country, Mum and Dad stepped in to help with childcare and, riddled with guilt at having to leave Josh each day, I was desperate to spend as much quality time with him as I was able. It meant that for me, like a lot of working parents, evenings, weekends and any holidays were precious and we made the most of our time together: bug hunting in the park, going on adventures, eating picnics, running around in the woods and watching movies. In fact, just *one* movie – *A Bug's Life*. I still know the entire script by heart nearly twenty years later!

We lived an ordinary little life.

A happy life.

As a toddler, Josh was inquisitive about the world, and my expertise on topics as diverse as space travel and spiders wasn't nearly enough to satisfy his thirst for knowledge. He had an insight that was as fascinating as it was alarming. His boredom threshold was low and, sadly, my need to work to put food on the table high – and so I devised an ingenious way to keep his brain occupied and his fingers busy by getting him to daily perform the job of 'peg sorting'. You are not familiar with this most important of chores? Let me enlighten you. I bought clothes pegs in an array of colours and would dump them in a pile on the kitchen floor along with old ice cream tubs. Then, I'd ask for Josh's help as I was *so* busy with other chores, would he possibly mind sorting out the pegs into colour groups for me? This simple task could buy me as much as half an hour – enough to get through a slew of emails or wash the dishes and give the kitchen a quick once over. He would sit diligently organising the pegs into colour groups and was always so proud to show me them sitting neatly in their ice cream tubs.

'Wow! Josh, thank you so much, that has saved me a job.'

He always looked delighted to have been of such use. Many of my friends and family thought it was such a neat idea that they too employed the 'peg sorting' chore as well, which miraculously needed doing on most days – I'm *still* puzzled as to how those darned pegs would get mixed up every evening just after Josh's bedtime . . .

Josh was smart and was able to outmanoeuvre me from a very young age. I was preparing dinner one day when he asked for a biscuit. I told him no, as it was close to suppertime and I didn't want him to spoil his appetite. He toddled off, but came back a minute later to say, 'Would *you* like a biscuit, Mum?'

'No, Josh, I wouldn't.'

I was puzzled until he said, 'I like it when you have a biscuit because you are such a good sharer!'

I still laugh about it now.

He also had an inability to lie. Now you might think this is a good thing – how many times do we press the importance of telling the truth on to our kids? There were times, however, when I wished this was not the case. And I would now like to apologise to the elderly lady who lived in the flat above who Josh and I met one day by the bins and to whom he said, 'Mummy said she wonders what your flat is like and that when you die we are going to cut a hole in our ceiling and put a ladder up through the floor, so we can have an upstairs, and get rid of all your old stuff.'

'Did you, Mandy?' came her understandably horrified reply.

'Well,' I took a deep breath, following my son's example for honesty, 'yes, but Josh is making it sound a lot more callous than I intended it . . .'

The irony is not lost on me that as Josh's depression took hold he became very good at lying.

'Is everything okay with you, Joshy?'

'Yes. Everything's fine . . .'

As a child, he was also very protective of us as a twosome. I still cringe to recall meeting a friend's boyfriend in the park who innocently asked, 'So, what do you like doing at weekends, Josh?'

Josh looked him in the eye and said, 'I like spending time with my mum on our own; just the two of us in the park or watching *Bug's Life* with no one else on the sofa talking to us or interrupting.'

The guy looked absolutely mortified! It was the fastest dash to the car park I have ever made.

I come from a large, close East End family where children are kings, the kind of household where all activity stops so a child can sing a song, recite a poem or tell us a snippet about their day, followed by rapturous applause. Joshy was no different in that everyone adored him. They still do. My grandparents were some of the first to pitch up at the hospital on the day he was born, with a miniature West Ham football kit to bestow upon 'the boy'. My parents, who had moved from London to the West Country, fell in love with him and remain so to this day. His scrawled stick men drawings were framed; his artwork plastered all over the kitchen cabinets and anecdotes (of interest to no one but his grandparents) were recounted down the telephone line to whichever friend, relative or unlucky salesperson happened to be calling.

I had always felt that coming from a large family gave me a wonderful safety net of support, and with this in mind, when Josh was two we moved to be closer to my parents and he thrived. He had an incredible vocabulary in which I took immense pride, watching him chat about anything and everything quite comfort-ably before he was even in school. This child was smart, nay gifted. The sky was the limit! I make no secret of the fact I used to lie in bed at night in our little flat, listening to his childhood snuffles of slumber, imagining all the wonderful things he might achieve. I was determined to work as hard as I could and encourage him every day to achieve whatever it might be that would make him happy.

Things changed when he started at nursery, removed for the first time from the bubble and safety of family life. He was one of those kids who didn't quite seem to fit at school. I noticed very early on a disconnect between his verbal acuity and his written ability. This was never more prominent than when I got home from my weekend job in a call centre and asked what he had been up to. He told me with energy and enthusiasm, 'Mum! We went on a boat and I helped put the spinnaker up and we sped up really fast and overtook three other crews and I got a medal!'

It sounded wonderful. He brought home his book of 'news' the following Monday and there was a vast, crudely drawn picture of a sail on the sea along with two words, each letter written inches high so they filled the page: 'Ma bot.' I asked Josh what it said and he said, 'It says "Me on the boat." That's my news!' He looked angry and frustrated, close to tears. This I understood, unable to imagine having all those thoughts and images in my head and not being able to put them down on paper.

Josh found reading and writing incredibly hard. This was odd for me as books had been my escape, my friends and my educa-tors for as long as I could remember. The day I was given my first library ticket in its little green cardboard holder and taught about the Dewey Decimal System is still one of my best ever. That library ticket and access to all those printed words changed my life. I kept in mind that he was still so very young and the last thing I wanted to do was put any undue pressure on my little boy, aware that everyone develops at different rates and that maybe he just hadn't found his stride yet. Not that Josh didn't love books; he did, and some of my favourite memories are of snuggling next to him before bedtime and working our way through Lemony Snicket's 'A Series of Unfortunate Events' together. This collection of books is among my most treasured possessions, each page crammed with memories so vivid that I only have to crack the spine at a particular page and I can feel his little body folded against mine, listening intently as I read aloud.

Josh was at the time unfortunate enough to have a teacher who felt the best thing for Josh's education was to sit him with his back to the rest of the class to help him '*concentrate*' and to '*stop him asking so many questions*'. I was shocked at her methods, but also completely ignorant of educational systems. I felt I had to trust her; she was highly regarded and I heard many parents extol her skill. She was the expert. Or so I thought.

I now wish I had listened to that voice of instinct that sat on my shoulder, telling me that to isolate a child who might be experiencing difficulty was the very worst thing possible. I wanted to know how best to help and encourage Josh and thought a firm diagnosis would be the way to do that, a springboard allowing us to figure out how best to educate him. He was then paraded in front of several experts and in due course given so many labels: dyslexia, dyspraxia. I went online and sifted through various definitions, ideas and suggestions and if anything I was more confused than ever. Josh's range of behaviours seemed to straddle so many different conditions. I thought he might be autistic, but that was ruled out by specialists with one telling me, 'No, Josiah isn't autistic. He's just a little complicated . . .' This I knew.

I believe the decline in Josh's mental health took root in the classroom at a young age, and, sadly, this is not unusual. A recent NHS report shared in the *Independent* stated: 'In a class of thirty children, four could be expected to be contending with emotional disorders, such as depression and anxiety, behavioural or hyperactive disorders that are impacting their well-being.'[6]

And this is not only a UK issue; in America it is reported that 'more than one in twenty US children and teens have anxiety or depression'.[7] These figures on both sides of the pond are as horrifying as they are sobering and I can't help but look beyond the numbers and picture the faces of children just like mine who are suffering right now as he did.

Josh found forming friendships hard, preferring the company of one or two rather than a large group, where I think he found the noise and multi-faceted interactions a little overwhelming. Was it any wonder when he wasn't allowed to sit with his peers or even face them? His isolation spilled over into sports and playtimes and I saw first hand how friendship groups made in the classroom bloomed in the playground, and how he was shunned by some of the other children. It tore at my heart. Even to think of it now is really painful. Josh was then, as he is now, a sweet, kind boy with a strong sense of justice. Mistreatment at the hands of his peers was something he found very hard to fathom. A boy was overheard saying some really horrible things to Josh. The head of school became involved and both boys were called before her. She told me that she asked Josh if he wanted the boy to get into trouble and he shook his head and said, 'No, I just want it to stop. I wish everyone could be kind.' She told me the perpetrator was simply delighted not to be receiving a punishment and wasn't in the least bit apologetic. She also said something that I recall even now. 'Today I can see the men these two boys will become and Josh is going to be a lovely citizen of the planet, kind. You should be very proud . . .'

And she was right, he is. And I am. Not that her endorsement was enough to ensure happy school days, and one of the biggest regrets of my life is that I left him in a school where he was labelled so definitively and marked by his peers at the age of three.

Three . . . Just a little baby really.

Josh, I now think, spent his school years (he left the school at eighteen) cowering under or hiding behind the labels that had been glued to him for life. They did him a great disservice, failed him. And I accept my part for not acting more decisively. For not having the courage to insist he change to one of the schools we visited, instead of leaving the decision to him. I should have taken the reins and insisted. I thought this autonomy when other aspects of his life were beyond his control was important, but I can see that I failed him too. His fear at the prospect of changing schools seemed at the time to outweigh the positives of shifting. If the guilt I feel about Josh's depression is a trifle, then his young age – spent at the mercy of this teacher – is the sponge layer. I still remember the day that particular educator sat me down and told me it was unlikely Josh would ever be able to write his own name. It's really hard to recall. I had taken the morning off work for the meeting, was anxious about my job and walked home in tears with a tangle of thoughts: *what the hell do I do now? Where do I go for help? And what does life look like for a boy like Josh who can't write his name?*

The picture she painted was about as far as it could be from the life I had envisaged for my little boy. From that day on my expectations and wants for Josh changed. Forget his being the best lawyer/doctor/poet/artist on the planet – I was now determined to try to ensure that if he ever had to fill out a form or sign something he would be able to do so without the excruciating awkwardness of not knowing how.

Josh proved her wrong, eventually. In fact, he proved us all wrong. Good Lord, he's even written half a book! With a combination of his incredible memory, speed of recollection, strong opinions and charm, he effectively buried his dyslexia under the proof of good grades and glowing school reports that extolled his politeness, razor-sharp sense of humour and enquiring mind.

This was pretty much the story of his whole school life, almost success by stealth. That was until a good teacher – no, a *great* teacher, an angel in fact, let's call her Dr P – told Josh, at the age of eleven, that he had a gift for Biological Sciences. She told him he could study it to the highest level if he wanted.

Her words lit something within him in a way that I had never seen. He felt excited about a future with Science as his chosen field of study. He explained to me how in every lesson he felt as if he already *knew* the subject, he just got it! And he spent the next few years devouring documentaries, books, anything he could on Biology and related topics. I remember at the age of eight he requested a copy of *Gray's Anatomy*, which he learned by heart, and even though he was only young he could talk with confidence about the human body, how it worked and why it went wrong. Dr P told us that Josh was always asking questions way beyond the scope of the lesson, some of them to degree level, showing insight and the natural ability of a curious mind in tune with the discipline. The irony is not lost on us that whilst he knows the physical being inside out and back to front, even more so now, the mental workings of the human brain have been a lot harder for him to master.

Dr P gave Josh a reason to walk with his shoulders back and his chin lifted for the first time ever. She was a great, great teacher who made him believe he could achieve something. I cannot think of her without a lump of raw emotion in my throat. This small cup of confidence from which he sipped had magical powers. Josh started to engage more in conversation; he laughed longer, walked taller and carried a new positive energy that was as infectious as it was exciting. She gave him the first helping of self-esteem he had ever been dished out at school – and most important, she gave him hope. I will forever be indebted to her and I hope she knows what a difference she made to our lives. I think of her often.

Despite Josh's sense of humour at home or when he was with me, where he was keen to express his comic views on things, he was not a jolly kid, not a joker or a jovial clown – quite the opposite. He was very young when daily he began to complain of aches in his groin/knees/wrists/elbows/neck. At first, with so many varied physical complaints, I suspected these protestations might be a ruse to try to escape being sent to school, but as he grew, it became clear to anyone who saw him that this was not the case. His stilted movement and grimacing expression put me in mind of my own childhood when, between surgeries and treatment for my dodgy pelvis, identified rather vaguely as a 'congenital defect', I would wake up and struggle to get going with joints that felt like they were on fire or throbbing with pain. For Josh too, the mornings were particularly bad and I can picture him walking slowly with stiff legs and the wince of an old man as he made his way down the stairs in his school uniform. He said it was difficult to play sport as his joints hurt so much after even minimal activity. My medicine for him was hot baths, cold compresses, the odd Ibuprofen and sofa rest. I didn't know what else to do. His symptoms were so vague and shifting.

'What hurts, Josh?'
'Everything.'
'But what hurts the most?'
'All of me.'

I took him to a GP who looked as perplexed as I felt by the wide range of aches and said it was most likely growing pains. I took some small relief from this, thinking that at least he would grow out of whatever it was. And it couldn't happen quickly enough. It felt like yet another boulder blocking his development.

If I look back to his early childhood, I can see that Josh always seemed a little sad, and this had been his manner since nursery school: a little reserved, a little lacking in confidence, stooped and reticent to try something new or join in. I had always been the child whose hand would shoot up to volunteer for anything, from an impromptu sing-song to taking the register to the office – I would jump from my seat with my hand pointing towards the asbestos ceiling, '*Me! Me! Oooh, pick me!*' Josh was the exact opposite. I noticed his anxiety increase in certain situations, like having to use a lift or interact with strangers:

> '*Go get a drink from the kiosk.*'
> '*I don't want to. Can you go, Mum?*'

> '*Give the money to the bus driver.*'
> '*I can't. I just can't. You do it.*'

> '*You've been invited to a birthday party.*'
> '*I don't actually have to go, do I?*'

I now recognise these traits as anxiety, but back then I thought it was just a little shyness that he could and most probably would overcome. Josh started to not want to go out at all. And in between my long working hours I tried to distract him from this seemingly melancholy state by thinking about what might make him feel better, even if it was just for a little while. I made every suggestion possible: *Shall we invite a friend for tea? How about a party? A playdate? Let's go for a walk! To the zoo! The cinema! A picnic! Shall we read a book? How about a trip to the seaside? Want to go and see Nanny and Grandad? We could stop off at ToysRUs?*

God, ToysRUs – even writing the name sends me into a cold sweat. I have lost count of the number of times, the wasted hours, when I traipsed around the cavernous store grabbing him bits of flimsy plastic-made crap, which he didn't really want and that I could ill afford, just trying to buy him a moment of joy. A distraction. But that was my life. I lived in that second, dancing in circles and jumping through hoops in an attempt to make everything a little bit better. The ridiculous thing, looking back, is that not only did I not know *how* to make things better, I didn't even know what I was trying to fix. I was a busy fool. A busy, exhausted fool, fuelled by emotion and a deep-seated desire to make everything better. I just didn't know how.

With the glorious benefit of hindsight, I can now see the parallel between my actions then and my actions in recent years. I think that from the day he was born I have been trying to help Josh find happiness, and I liken my behaviour to that of a sweeper in curling, toiling to remove any and all obstacles to ensure a smooth glide path, and I believed this to be the right course of action. I laugh now at my naivety, the fact that I once believed this to be possible without comprehending that his mental state would not and could not be healed by a nice day out, a good dinner or a trip to the cinema.

Not that I think my actions were entirely futile; I can think of times when I have had some small measure of success, moments when my kindness and love have served as a welcome diversion, like a warm bath for an aching back, only enjoyable momentarily, and entirely pointless for a long-term fix, but pleasant nonetheless. These small acts of kindness, like full stops, are necessary to give structure, a break, a change in tone or direction, but I now also know they do not and cannot alter the narrative that, for my son, unhappiness has, for much of his life, been his default state. I was waiting for the time Josh might present as truly happy! And I told myself it would happen when he finished that school year . . . when we went on holiday . . . Christmas time . . . when he could ride a bike . . . when he reached ten . . . thirteen . . . sixteen . . . eighteen . . . passed his exams . . . made a team . . . went to university . . . I still do this.

I'd watch the other boys in his class running around the playground, a little band of mates, a club, a gang, and I wished that Joshy knew the code, how to gain entry, but he didn't and I couldn't help him. On the rare days when work allowed and I got to collect him from school, I hated to hear the casual conversation between the other parents and carers who seemed to know each other very well and whose kids played together regularly, strengthening the bonds:

'Football was fun this week!'

'It was. Whose turn is it to pick up for swimming?'

'Mine. Are we still all on for the picnic?'

And I knew the alienation and awkwardness I felt, trying to be part of the mums' club, was only a flicker of how Josh felt on a daily basis. And again my heart broke for him. These encounters shored up the wall of guilt over which I had to hurdle each time I left our little flat to go to work. I began to question: would Josh's life be happier, easier if I didn't work? But this immediately threw up questions – what about *my* life and how on earth would we live? I still wanted to be the best example to him I could be.

I saw many red flags in Josh's behaviour and hated the pattern-setting, but I honestly did not know who to discuss this with or how best to help him. I did speak to my brothers, who assured me Josh was a great kid and would be fine, my Auntie Josie, who pointed out that when you were super smart or a little bit different, life was not always easy, and my grandparents, who dismissed my concerns altogether and told me not to worry. I mentioned my concerns too to my GP, more as an aside, that I was a little worried about Josh.

'I feel guilty about working such long hours but I don't have any choice. We are only just about managing. But my son is full of aches and pains every single day. Plus he seems reserved, awkward and anxious . . .' I swallowed.

41

'Ah, well it wouldn't do for us all to be the same,' came his rather fey, ineffective response. I didn't confess to the fleeting thought that if it meant my child had an easier ride through school, part of me wished we *were* all the same – what wouldn't I give to see Josh huddling with the gang, kicking a ball about, laughing . . .

My parents' love and support has always been unconditional and naturally they were the people I could most easily confide in. But of course they could only see any issues through the gauze of their devout love for Josh.

'He's a wonderful child. He'll be fine. You need to not pass on your anxiety to him. He'll be fine, Mandy, you'll see . . .'

I knew this in part was right, I didn't want to pass any of my anxiety on to him, thinking that if he was aware of my concerns this might only add to his worries or at worst, legitimise his anxiety. And so I worked hard at telling Josh and myself that everything was going to be okay. I wanted so desperately to believe it. He was still only a little boy and I clung to this firm-held belief that it would be all right in the end, we would battle through somehow, together.

Chapter Four

JOSH

'YEAH, JOSH, WHAT IS WRONG WITH YOU?'

'If a man does not keep pace with his companions, perhaps it is because he hears a different drummer. Let him step to the music which he hears, however measured or far away.'

Henry David Thoreau

I suspect that like most people, memories of my babyhood are sketchy.

I know that in my baby years I lived in and around London, but can only remember living in Bristol, where we moved before I was two. It's a city I have always loved. My hometown.

I'm not sure if it is my earliest memory or whether it's a tale I have been told and along with photographic evidence have woven into my memory, but I picture myself walking along the side of a road in Clifton, Bristol, and I'm wearing reins – those little baby harnesses that seem somehow caring and yet a little cruel at the same time. I know I must have been very young as I recall being very close to the floor, no more than a couple of feet or so, hard to imagine as a grown-up.

I don't know where we were heading, I don't know who is on the other end of the reins, but I can well remember that feeling of wanting to run and being held back, straining against the leash, frustrated, unaware that this state of affairs might be for my own safekeeping.

It's a feeling that has become familiar to me throughout my life.

That frustration – feeling like I want to run but am anchored – has in fact been a constant. It's lessening with age a bit but even now if I am forced to sit in a confined or crowded space or when boredom creeps in, the desire to bolt is strong. And this was never more the case than when in school. An environment that didn't suit me. I would gaze at the window like a prisoner longing for the outside world, mentally counting down the minutes. Mum used to say I had ants in my pants, but if this was true, I also had ants in my brain, scurrying this way and that, making concentrating nigh on impossible.

I listen to Mum talking with such energy, such joy about giving birth to me and I almost dare not tell her that I often think about the time before I was born, that nothingness, and how attracted I am to the idea of that perfect state of non-consciousness that has for me in the last few years been the state to which I wanted to return.

She talks about how *happy* she was to become a mum, how *happy* she was to spend time with me, and again it's a hard truth that the state of happiness to which she refers has been elusive my whole life. I used to think I wasn't capable of feeling happy, even doubting the existence of the phenomena that others were so readily able to describe. Now? I'm not so sure. I see glimpses of it. I feel the beginnings of it. And this gives me hope.

As a small child I was puzzled by all the minutiae that my peers seemed obsessed with. I used to look at the giggling kids who lapped the playground hand in hand and wonder why they didn't get how serious this whole business of life was! I spent most of my time looking up, concerned with why we were and how we got here. Surely I couldn't have been the only one with bigger things to worry about than Play-Doh and plastic dinosaurs (although I do really, really like dinosaurs!).

The things that fascinated my peers felt to me a bit pointless. I couldn't share their enthusiasm for football, couldn't understand why they were so keen to run around after a small white ball when there were mysteries of the universe to figure out. What did they mean we revolved around the sun?! How was wind made? Who made all the rules and what if they were wrong?

I remember staring at a teacher who was trying to make us repeat vowel sounds and looking over her shoulder at a poster of the planets and thinking, *Forget that! Tell us about the solar system! What are planets made of? How did they get there? What are those rings around Saturn? And is there life on Mars?*

It's a difficult thing to admit that at nursery and primary school it felt like I spoke a different language, was from a foreign land and no matter how much I wanted to join in, be one of the gang, I didn't know how. I tried, but it didn't get me very far. At some point I stopped trying. My self-imposed exile fitted the agenda, I suppose. People left me to it and that was probably a relief, although a relief that did little to curb the loneliness.

Primary school was tough, frightening, overwhelming and it's fair to say I hated nearly all of it. It's hard to think of a good day. I used to climb reluctantly from the car and wish I didn't have to, wanting to stay in the car or go with Mum to work, anything other than have to walk into that classroom for the whole day. It felt like a punishment. I recall one particular teacher on a day when I was struggling to do as she asked losing her temper, her face so close to mine that I held my breath as she screamed, 'Why can't you write your name? Why can't you? Everyone else can do it!' She pointed to my classmates.

My heart raced. I felt sick, embarrassed, exposed and stupid, really stupid. I can recall that feeling clearly even now nearly two decades later. It damaged me. I remember looking around the room at the kids who looked like me but were not *like* me and I thought yeah, why can't you do it, Josh? What is wrong with you?

Her anger and frustration were clearly and publicly expressed and it was as scary as it was humiliating. I shall never forget it. Her pitch, her expression. I can only assume that she felt my lack of ability reflected on her in some way, but it was horrific, abusive and, I can now see, totally misplaced. As an adult, I can't imagine doing that to a child: in fact, I can't imagine doing that to an adult.

The only small sparks of joy in my life came from interacting with my grandad, an engineer, and helping him build or repair things in his workshop or making bonfires around which we'd sit, and talking to my Great-Uncle Pete on my dad's side, who was an environmental scientist. He taught me about the significance of ocean temperature. These practical, intelligent grown-ups held my interest and I wanted to know more of what they knew.

Mum tried to distract me from the dread of Monday morning that loomed large over my weekends, casting a shadow over every activity and even the best of days. The thought of going back to school ticked loudly like a metronome, getting faster and faster as Sunday night drew closer. I remember she bought me an iPod when I was about seven and told me it would help me escape; that music could take me anywhere I wanted to go at any time.

That small, slim rectangular device was indeed a portal into another world, and the world of music is still one into which I often tumble, although in those days I listened to Gorillaz and Green Day, whereas now it's more likely to be Mall Grab or Denis Sulta and a lot, lot louder. Music is my escape and fires my imagination like no other medium.

I tried again to explain to Mum only recently how I longed for that time before birth and saw the distress flicker across her face, distress she tries and often fails to hide.

She asked me recently, as she often does, to explain, to try and help her understand, and so I told her this: 'Existence is exhausting, you experience and process one moment in time and immediately there's another one to be processed. It's an endless, daunting, relentless cycle going on forever till we die. I think the closest we can ever get to Nirvana is that infinite nothingness of before we were rudely ripped into consciousness.'

She cried and muttered, '*What the hell, Josh?*'

And here we are: her trying to make everything all right and not knowing how, and me trying every day to process wave after wave of intrusive thoughts and stave off this permanent state of exhaustion whilst doing my very best to fit in.

If I think about it, this is how it has always been: a bad day at school might mean a new toy to add to the large collection of crap I didn't play with, and I suppose it did lift my mood momentarily, but was no solution. The realisation that this has been my whole life is frustrating and upsetting. I would have thought that a) she'd have got it by now and b) I might have figured out a way to stop or alter this thought process, because in all honesty I'm bloody knackered.

Photographs

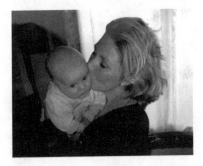

Me aged twenty-eight with Josh at ten weeks' old, living in a damp house running alive with rats that nested in the cupboards, but even that couldn't dent the joy I felt at having, against all the odds, become a mum.

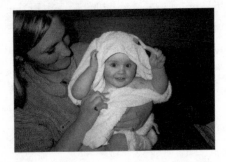

Josh at six months. Bath time was always a drawn-out, splashy affair that ended with both the bathroom and us entirely soaked.

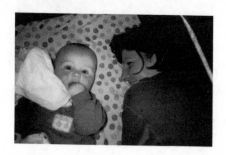

Josh with Nanny Annie, who used to spend hours staring at him, totally in love . . . She still does!

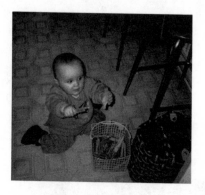

Mandy: Visiting Great-Nanny and Great-Grandad in Rainham, Essex. Josh of course headed straight for the pegs and very kindly sorted them for them!

Josh: I can't remember at what age I became aware that peg counting was just a huge diversion, but I liked doing it anyway, so . . . win win! We still refer to pointless chores as peg counting.

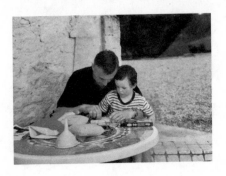

Josh: I was aged three in this one. It's me and my grandad Ken. He was showing me something or playing a game. I do remember this summer and I know I was happy.

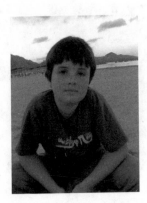

Josh: I'm eight here. Mum took the picture on the beach in Puerto Pollença, Mallorca. I think this expression sums me up at this age: a half-smile, even though we were on holiday and that was nice; I was still quite anxious.

Chapter Five

Amanda

'The world is his oyster!'

'I cannot fix on the hour, or the spot, or the look, or the words, which laid the foundation. It is too long ago. I was in the middle before I knew that I had begun.'

Jane Austen

I fell in love when Josh was eight.

It was and still is a wonderful surprise to me that having vowed to stay single, smarting from my short-lived marriage and with emotional bruises that ran deep, Cupid, despite my protestations to the contrary, was taking aim. Even if I had been interested in diving back into the dating pool, as a working single mum with no social life it was hard to see how I could find a partner, let alone make time for them alongside the work and parenting that filled my days. Friends had over the years tried to introduce me to 'this really, really great guy!' Their offers, well meant, were always politely refused. When I said I wasn't looking for anyone, happy in my single status,

I wasn't joking. Josh and his well-being were my priority and to introduce someone else would, I knew, alter the dynamic of our little family. This would be the case whether it worked out or not. And frankly it was a risk I was unwilling to take.

A fundamental rule of my parenting then and now was to promise Josh I would never make a decision that I thought might be harmful to him and I would only ever try to do things that would make our life better, even if this wasn't always immediately obvious. I explained, for example, that if I worked late or long hours, either at my main office job or at one of the other evening and weekend jobs in call centres and cleaning I took to supplement my income, I wasn't abandoning him, but was instead putting the graft in to make sure we kept the roof over our head, and if he was missing me, he could be darned sure I was missing him right back. If I said 'no' to something it would be with good reason: either that thing might be harmful – *'Can I drink this aftershave, Mum?'* – or, as in the case of *'Can we go to the Kennedy Space Center next Thursday?'* I could not afford it, plus it was a long, long way away.

I met Simeon, a soldier and the dad of Ben, Josh's school friend, at a school rugby match. He was a kind, funny, loyal man, who asked questions about Josh, but was reassuringly unfazed by the fact that I, like him, was a single parent, and it gave me the confidence to leap.

Simeon saw Josh and me as a package. I felt happy in his company, very happy, and I liked the way he treated my son. He didn't rush to befriend him, and let Josh dictate the pace. It felt nice to have someone to share life with, the good and the bad, and to have another grown-up on hand to sense-check my decisions was something wonderful. Plus, my beloved grandma fell in love with him too. I think it was something to do with the fact that he was a soldier and the uniform, even in the later stages of her life when her mind had dulled a little, evoked fond memories of her own wartime love . . . and that was all the approval I needed.

I decided to take the plunge, knowing I wanted a future with this man in it, and eventually he and his son, Ben, merged their little duo with ours and hey presto! I suddenly had two sons and the husband I had told myself for years I did not want. I knew that forming a new family would not be without its challenges, but it would be a lie to say that I didn't consider the fact that in my opinion, a stable, smart man like Simeon might just be the kind of ally that a boy like Josh needed. Josh's dad is great and has been ever-present in Josh's life, but it was the day-to-day living that I knew Simeon would make a difference to.

It was around this time that Josh finally received a diagnosis for all the aches and pains that had dogged him for years: Elhers Danlos Syndrome. I had never heard of it and didn't know whether to be delighted to finally know what we were dealing with or devastated to read about the condition. It is essentially a connective tissue disorder characterised by joint hypermobility and there is no cure, but his symptoms can be managed. It can be hereditary or can appear for the first time. Having read the symptoms of EDS, which can include spontaneous abortion, I wonder if I have it too as I have had at least ten miscarriages that I know of, plus there is my mystery pelvic and back pain and subsequent surgeries throughout my youth, as well as my extra double-jointed bendy wrists and fingers. However, I have not yet had a formal diagnosis.

Ignorant of the condition, I spent the month or so after Josh's diagnosis glued to a computer screen reading of the most extreme cases and crying myself to sleep. It is a syndrome with a vast spectrum of severity and Josh suffers in the mid region of the scale, enough to wake with his overextended joints – wrists, groin, shoulders, lower back – in various states of pain that range from mild to severe. No wonder he was fed up. I know it isn't easy and on bad days even the most basic of tasks presents a challenge. For him to play sport, for example, means the next day he will be unable to move, and getting to sleep in a comfortable, non-painful position is often impossible, meaning his sleep is disrupted every single night. This is a torture in itself.

Throughout Josh's school life, Simeon encouraged him to try various sports, to find the things he was able to do with the least amount of discomfort the next day. And try he did. It tore at my heart to see him tackle a sport or activity with such enthusiasm and then watch him the following morning walking slowly, stiff-limbed down the stairs with his face contorted. Waving Josh off to school every day knowing he was going to have to hurdle over dyslexia, anxiety and now the debilitating Elhers Danlos whilst struggling to fit in with his peers, took its toll. The temptation was to wrap him in cotton wool and keep him safe and sound at home, but I knew this was not the way to build resilience in him. But I'll admit it was a struggle, and went against my maternal instinct to make him comfortable and let him stay at home out of harm's way.

Whilst there were many aspects of Josh's school life that were a cause for concern, ironically in the end his academic ability was not to be one of them. Despite his rather shaky start when the prognosis looked just about as bad as it could be, Josh turned out to be more than able, smart in fact. I stole a phrase from my parents and told Josh very early on that 'his normal was his normal' and no matter how hard he found trying to learn with dyslexia, he needed to find some coping strategies and figure out how it was going to work for him. And to his credit, he did. Watching him do his homework was painstaking, and it wasn't helped by the fact that my other son, Ben, was often working on similar if not the same assignments, and would rattle through them, free then to hit the PlayStation. Of course it wasn't Ben's fault, but nevertheless it was a bit like holding a mirror up to Josh's inability and that inevitably caused tensions.

Many a night Josh would be at the table near tears, struggling to write a sentence and get the words, which rattled around inside his head, down on paper. It was a long time coming, but gradually he mastered the art of reading and writing. Even now he might not always perfect the spelling and progress is still slow, but he can certainly write his name. His incredible memory became like a superpower, enabling him to watch a documentary or listen to something, and then repeat it verbatim – a neat trick when it came to exams, which he coasted through. He was offered a scribe for exams, but interestingly, such was his mistrust of the educational hierarchy, as well as being unconvinced that they would interpret his words or thoughts exactly, that he preferred to rely on a little extra time and his own (almost illegible) handwriting.

Josh rarely revised, confident that the facts were locked down in his memory. As he progressed through school and was able to choose subjects that favoured his learning style with fewer essays and more practical assessments, he flew. He continued to do what worked for him, listening to excerpts read from textbooks or watching lectures, able to remember the information. His intelligence was in every sense his saving grace, his intellect the thing of which he was most proud, and he was determined not to let his dyslexia be a barrier to success. I took great comfort from this and knew that with the determination he showed he could reach for the stars. I remember sitting with him on the sofa and looking up lists of all the people who had excelled despite suffering with dyslexia, people who didn't necessarily have qualifications but who seemed to be risk-takers and even some who saw the condition as a gift, enabling them to look at the world in a different way.

He excelled in the sciences, with Biology being his great love. His school reports were always the same – top grades for the subjects where he could tackle the examination with a multiple-choice exam and coursework and not so fabulous grades for anything in which he had to write a long essay or read a book – *quelle surprise*. This was of course partly down to his dyslexia, but also because Josh very much gives attention and time to the things he enjoys and that which he doesn't takes a back seat. Not that we cared, we didn't want him to be great at everything and there was no pressure to excel at anything, we just wanted him to be reaching his potential and were more than content that he had found one thing he loved. We were still intent on keeping 'happy as the goal' and tried not to overwhelm the boys with pressure. Every term it felt like we made small progress and that was enough.

Simeon and I were happy. We lived in a little army house with a leaky roof, our boys were settled and we were deeply in love. Life was good.

At sixteen Josh sat his GCSEs and for the first time I knew what it felt like to be one of those mums in the chattering club, the ones who were keen to regale the details of their son's sporting achievement, the ones who wanted to laugh over a latte about their kid's latest accolade, and it felt brilliant! Josh excelled in the exams, securing 'A' grades in just about every subject. I wanted to rent a billboard and plaster them on it. I was so proud, knowing how important a win it was for Josh and in truth delighting at what felt like a turning point. For the first time I took my foot off the pedal of concern and allowed myself to believe that Josh was finally, finally within grabbing distance of that happy life I wished for him. This was so much more than his nan and grandad, blinkered by their love for him, framing his stick man drawing; this was a national exam body giving him the stamp of approval that put him on a par with or even ahead of the national average and we were over the moon – this for a boy who had struggled to make the grade his whole young life.

I have some lovely memories of this time, some funny ones too – including the day Josh came down the stairs with a look of worry to say he had forgotten to bring home a vital DT (design and technology) project which he needed to work on over the half-term holiday. There seemed to be only one solution: to break into his school and grab the project! I think Josh thought I was joking until only half an hour later we were outside the school annex. After rattling a few windows and noticing the burglar alarm blinking in the corner of the building, we decided to try to gain lawful entry. A very kind caretaker agreed to open one of the doors so we could access the corridor but made us promise not to enter any of the classrooms, with their dangerous equipment – stuff like scissors and laminating machines . . . We both promised with our fingers crossed behind our backs.

Josh knew a way to the DT room and we snuck along in the semi darkness through a rabbit warren of corridors and a huge storage space until we were where we needed to be.

'Right, Mum,' Josh whispered, 'can you use your phone to take photos of the posters on the wall' – a quick glance told me there were many, giving hints and tips on how to do the best project and a few health and safety rules – 'while I find my project.'

It sounded like a plan and I eagerly whipped out my phone and spent at least ten minutes photographing the posters as best I could, making sure they were straight, legible and in focus. At one point we heard footsteps above and both dived under a workbench holding our breath. I was trying to figure out how I would justify being discovered hiding under the table with my son during the half-term break and could only think that they might rescind my invitation to have drinks and a mince pie with the Head and his wife over the festive period. Not that I was too bothered, I hate mince pies. Eventually Josh found his project and we legged it out of the building and into the car, laughing.

It was when we got home and told Simeon of our breaking and entering adventure that I asked Josh what I should do with all the photographs he had asked me to take.

'Anything you like,' came his nonchalant reply. 'I don't actually need them. I just couldn't think how else to occupy you for ten minutes and as there weren't any pegs that needed sorting into colours . . .'

Busted.

It still makes me laugh to this day – not only the fact that I took my role so very seriously, but also that Josh waited nearly two decades to take his revenge.

For Simeon and me, the period between the boys taking their GCSEs and their A level exams was one of glorious complacency. You know that incredible feeling when a worry is lifted from you and you feel free? It was exactly that. I slept better, functioned better and for the first time Simeon and I chatted about things other than our concerns over Josh on our evening walk. I think I only fully realised that I lived with this baseline worry about Josh when it was lifted and I felt the difference. The future looked like a rosy place. My writing had taken off and it was around this time that I published my third book, *Clover's Child*.

Both Ben and Josh were fabulous kids, and at nearly seventeen were shaping up to be fabulous men. Ben had set his heart on a career in the military and had identified his route for the next couple of years. We loved their company and each grew in ways that gave hints as to all that lay ahead. Ben was sporty and sociable, never happier than when out with his mates, and during this time of what I now see as 'respite' Josh seemed to have a contentment about him that was wonderful. Simeon's career was going in the right direction and he had been posted to Army HQ. Having completed over thirteen tours in some dusty and dangerous places, he was now based in Andover working on a project overhauling all the specialist equipment that had been utilised on active service. It might have meant some overnight separations, but it was a darned sight safer than Afghanistan.

I often think back to this time and wonder what I should have done differently. It's a horrible thought that maybe during this relaxed period, when I slept for a sound eight hours every night, I wasn't paying close enough attention, unaware of what lay in wait for our family – and, more importantly, what lay in wait for Josh.

He sat mock A levels aged seventeen and repeated the pattern set by his GCSEs, sailing through them with a clutch of A's and A*s. This was it! Our boy was going to go to university and he was going to grab armfuls of life and run with it, just as I had always pictured for him. With his mock results under his belt, offers from universities flooded in and Josh found himself in a wonderful position, torn as to which to accept. All were offers to study his beloved Biology and dependent on his final grades, the exams he would take in the summer. He finally made the decision, accepting an offer from St Andrews with Exeter as a backup. Simeon and Josh took a boys' trip, visiting each place and looking at accommodation before sampling brunch. It was nothing but exciting! The whole family was ecstatic for him. Imagine, our Josh was going to study at one of these prestigious seats of learning – he had done it. The world was his oyster. His promising future felt like vindication, as though finally, finally it was Josh's time. We pressed the point that he could start over, a new beginning. Never again would he sit with his back to the class – and I for one could not wait to watch him bloom.

Chapter Six

Josh

'Falling through the cracks'

'And yet to every bad there is a worse.'

Thomas Hardy

My Elhers Danlos diagnosis didn't really change much for me. Not as much as I thought or hoped it would. How my body worked and all the physical limitations were exactly as they had always been. I ached each morning and was in pain most nights and sports were still a challenge, which made life at a very sporty school difficult. The colder months were particularly tough, waking most mornings with random pains and feeling like I needed WD-40 in my knees and usually having to 'thaw them out' before attempting stairs. The main difference being I now had a hook with a label beneath it upon which to hang my symptoms and quirks.

Big deal. As my mum has always said, 'Your normal is your normal, right?' And she is right; my normal is my normal, no matter how abnormal it might appear to others.

Having Elhers Danlos was really just another change in my life that I chalked up to experience and tried to carry on with. It was just another piece of the jigsaw that made up the whole, less than perfect, slightly dissatisfying picture of me. There had been other changes to deal with during my formative years. Not least of which was when I was about eight and Mum decided to change the status quo of our family and marry my friend's dad. Yep, that went down well at school, as you can imagine. Mum and Simeon made out to be mates and no more than that; I can now see this was for our benefit, taking things slowly so as not to frighten me or my friend (now brother) Ben.

But this Hartley/Prowse merger was big news to me, a kid who had not considered other people might come and live under our roof, and it was, as I hinted, even bigger news in the school community, so much so that a member of staff saw fit to sit me down and ask, 'So, what's happening with your mum and Ben's dad then?'

It's only as an adult I can see how bloody crap this was; a grown woman fishing for gossip. These whispers were yet another aspect that made me feel a little different from my peers, but though the subject matter was no doubt humorous fodder for them, I had the last laugh because at the end of the day, I got Simeon.

I can't deny I was at first suspicious of the man and his motives, only able to see my mum as just that: my mum. The idea that she might also be a wife, a colleague, a sister, a daughter, a friend and the many other roles she fulfils did not occur to me – why would it? Simeon gradually morphed into her boyfriend, and then became her husband, facts that both horrified and delighted me. I looked forward to having him around, liked his willingness to play video games, an area in which Mum fell well short, but I was also fearful of the unknown. He started for me as an acquaintance, then turned into a friend and a father, and I can now say that he is the person who has got my back, someone I rely on 24/7, who is there for me no matter what and who has never given up on me, even when I tried to push him and everyone else away. He is thoughtful, calm and quiet in a crisis, whereas Mum has a tendency to lose it. Her crying has never added anything positive to a moment of high drama, and right off it seemed Simeon felt the same way; we would exchange a look and it made me feel like he got it. We still do that. It's nice.

As a little boy, if I had a nightmare, which was fairly often, he would sit on the floor and talk quietly to me until I went back to sleep, trying to supplant the images of monsters and impending apocalypse with memories of day trips, funny stories, anything to quell the demons that dogged me during sleep. And when as an adult I wanted to die, trying to make the choice between staying or ending it all, he sat on the floor of my bedroom and talked quietly to me until I fell asleep, trying to supplant my emptiness with substance, my despair with hope. His support has always been physical, mental, financial, emotional and unwavering.

He in fact is one of the reasons that I didn't take my own life.

I hope he knows this.

When he and Mum first got together, I both liked and hated having him and Ben in the house, depending entirely on my mood. It wasn't always easy. There were times when I missed my mum's undivided attention, but also there was the old safety in numbers thing, and to be part of a family of four was naturally a lot more reassuring than when there was only two of us. It gave me confidence to know that if one of us fell through the cracks, there were three people in the wings ready to pull them out. I guess at that time I already suspected that if anyone was going to fall through the cracks it would be me. Simeon helped me with my schoolwork and, like Mum, told me that whilst school might not be for me, what came next would be a revelation.

'Imagine, Josh, being at university and only studying the one subject that you love!'

This caught my imagination. Even at that young age, I couldn't wait. I decided I would immerse myself in the world of Biology and never have to dodge cross-country again. It would be bloody brilliant.

With Simeon's encouragement, my confidence at school grew and academically I soared. I might not have made the sports teams, but I had found my place in the science faculty. And it was a place I was happy to be. It felt like home.

They had been together for a couple of years when Mum gave up her job to write a book. She had always been a bookworm, something my dyslexic brain struggled to relate to, but I didn't realise quite how strong her passion for writing was. I don't think any of us could have predicted how this one simple act would change our lives. She has written over twenty-five novels since. I know that when she was writing her first book around 2011 and we were down to one income, things were tough. I could sense the tension in the air and heard her and Simeon talking in low tones around the kitchen table about money, or rather the lack of it. Neither of them addressed Ben or me directly on the subject, which was unsettling, but I remember feeling guilty if they gave me spending money or treated us. I might have only been young, but I recognised and appreciated that Simeon was not only encouraging me to follow a path that might make me happy, but my mum too.

We might not have had a lot of money, but life was looking up.

Buoyed up by my academic success, I agreed to enter a public speaking competition called 'Gabblers' where entrants from local schools had to write and learn a speech to be read out loud to all other competitors and a committee on a monthly basis. As reading the piece was so difficult for me, I would get someone to read it aloud a few times, enabling me to memorise it. My fear at being the boy sitting with his back to the class and my desire to be like everyone else reared its head, and so that everyone would think I was reading the words from the page, I would hold the paper and let my eye follow the text while speaking aloud. It took all of my courage. Not only did I have the fear of my dyslexia being publicly revealed, but interacting with strangers in the 'Gabblers' competition was also challenging for me, causing my anxiety to flare. I think I chose to do something so difficult to prove to myself and others that I was as capable as the next guy.

The grand 'Gabblers' finale was a black-tie affair with special invites sent out to parents and even the head of school. I was expected to write and present a speech on a given subject. I was randomly given the title 'Street Cred'. I was shit scared and so nervous beforehand, unsure how I would manage to stand and speak with conviction. One positive was that I had always been more comfortable talking to a large group of people than I was in a one-to-one situation. In fact, the larger the group the easier I found it. This was quite at odds with my preference to socialise in smaller groups, but when it came to 'performing', the lack of intimacy in a larger group was, for me, preferable. This is still the case to a degree. On this particular night, however, I nearly bottled it a few times and right before I stood up to speak I was not sure I could go through with it. But then they were calling my name and someone clapped and there I was at the lectern with the paper in my hand. A combination of nerves and dyslexia meant it could have been written in any language – not that it mattered; I had learned it by heart.

I took my time, trying not to look at the expectant faces of my parents and grandparents in the crowd, and did my best to blank out the room full of people. I took a deep breath, coughed to clear my throat and read aloud the title, 'Street Cred'; I then went off-piste, looked up and followed this immediately with the line 'Oh, the irony . . .'

And that was it, everybody laughed, laughed loudly! And they listened intently, waiting to hear what I said next. I spoke with conviction and was motivated by the looks of pride on the faces of those who knew and loved me. It felt brilliant. I won 'Best on the Night' for my speech and that was a pretty good feeling.

The head of school came up to me at the end of the night and shook my hand. He smiled and said, 'Well I never, Josiah, who knew you could do that?'

I looked him in the eye and thought about the years I had spent in his school, hiding away, never given a chance to shine, all because I couldn't catch a bloody ball or sprint over a line.

'*I* did, sir,' I replied. '*I* knew I could do that.'

He was seemingly at a loss as to how to reply.

It was the start of a very positive period for me. I was in my late teens and life felt full of possibilities.

Like my GCSEs, the exams taken at sixteen years of age, my results for the mock A levels, which are required for university entrance, were good, very good in fact. I felt a little smug, but also relieved and excited at what the future might hold, confident that results like these could be my ticket anywhere. Mum had always, in my moments of low mood or simply when I was reflecting, told me that I shouldn't take things to heart – so what if I wasn't that sporty? And that the main problem was that it was not my time – everyone had their time and mine was yet to come.

I believed her, and when she explained that whilst it might sound great to be one of the 'in crowd', did I *actually* want to be one of those people who could proudly announce that their school days were the best days of their lives? I mean, think about it, who wants to peak at fifteen? And how the hell do you top it or match it during the remaining sixty or so years? This thought gave me solace and I waited patiently for 'my time' to arrive. I didn't know for sure, but as I thought about heading off to university . . . it felt like my time might be right around the corner.

With my applications to various universities fired off and with letters of recommendation from my tutors to accompany them, offers to study, based on my mock results, came in thick and fast. It was the first time in my life that I felt parity with the kids who played for the A team. In fact, no, it was bigger than that, I felt parity with the whole fucking universe! Leading universities wanted me. Me! Josiah Hartley, the boy who would never write his name. I wanted to climb to the top of the school chapel and wave those offer letters from the roof whilst shouting, 'Fuck you all! Look what I got!'

I accepted places at St Andrews as my first choice, followed by Exeter, and started to picture myself walking the streets and visiting the bars, thinking of the incredible opportunity, finally able to shake off my old skin and start afresh in a new city with new experiences, new friends and a new beginning. I began to go out more in Bristol, enjoying the fantastic social life on offer, which centred mainly on the bars, pubs and clubs of Clifton. I think in part my newfound confidence was down to the fact that I had a future partly mapped out and it was one I was proud of: university and degree success. How hard could it be?

In this brief period of time, life was good, or at least life was better.

I knew, of course, that in the run-up to the actual exams I had to study to achieve the results on which my offers from St Andrews and Exeter were dependent. Weirdly, for someone who at this time had almost zero confidence in himself, this felt like a box-ticking exercise. I believed the required grades to be well within my grasp and I can honestly say that I was not overly fazed. I listened to the constant narcissistic chatter in the corridors, boys and girls alike, discussing the pressure, the demands, the incessant nagging from parents who demanded and then demanded more, desperate for their prodigies to excel and win, win, win – and don't even start on the stress!

I remained silently thankful that whilst Mum and Simeon encouraged me, I, like my brother Ben, were pretty much given free rein: studying was up to us and our choices were ours to make.

Not that they didn't then impress the consequences of those choices upon us, trying to navigate in the gentlest way possible. But the knuckle-clenching, pasty-faced, hollow stares of my peers who were wrecks, pushed at home, pushed at school and who seemed utterly terrified of failing? Let's just say I was very glad I was not one of them. I think it was the first time I became fully aware of how Mum and Simeon parented us. If my classmates' parents had them in a half nelson, mine in contrast had a hand placed gently on our shoulders. And I was grateful for it.

So with only the A level exams as the final hurdle, I knew it would not be enough to use my innate knowledge and charm to make my way through the trial. To get first-class grades and secure a place at my desired university would require the detail that came with study. I needed to be word perfect. And I was determined not to ruin this chance. I drew up a plan, deciding what to study on what day and I stuck it on the wall. I bought revision guides that I would go over at my own pace, more to test my knowledge and practise my précised responses than anything else. And with music growing ever more important to me, I pulled together a couple of playlists, one for studying and one for listening to when not studying. I dusted off the desk in my room and put the obligatory bottle of water within reach. I was set and ready to go. This work, this application to my subjects, was the final piece of the jigsaw. All I had to do was finish off a piece of coursework, revise, take the exam and this would see me over the line. I could then pack a bag and go seek my future.

Easy.

I was at the highest point mentally that I had ever been and I was ready, more than ready.

And then everything changed, and it occurred almost without warning.

Something very peculiar happened to me. I am still, even today with the benefit of a few years' reflection, genuinely at a loss as to how best to describe this peculiar thing. It's difficult, but I hope I can convey all I need to by the phrase I have chosen, which is this:

MY BRAIN SWITCHED OFF.

That's it. That's what happened.

I don't recall the exact day or minute, but I know it felt as if it happened in an instant. I sat at my well-ordered desk and opened a textbook to read up on coursework. After about an hour or so, I realised I had read the same page over and over, and each time it was as if it was the first time I had read it. And even after reading it repeatedly, none of it had stuck in my mind. Me, Josiah Hartley, who had sailed through the topic, who could recite whole textbooks of facts and information – I could not retain one single word. And *worse* than that, I could barely remember the first thing about any of the subjects of which my knowledge had been described as encyclopaedic. Nothing. Nothing at all.

It was like being given a book in a foreign language and one you are inadvertently holding upside down – not one word made sense. Or like being put in a network of tunnels and spun around so you don't know which way is up or even what direction you are walking in. Or like trying under pressure to remember the combination code that unlocks everything and not even remembering what a combination code is.

It was as if my brain were Teflon and everything I threw at it slid off without leaving a mark. And everything I had known had been syphoned out and replaced with goo.

I felt like I had run into a wall at speed.

I felt like my skull had been cleaved open.

My eyes were heavy and my head ached.

My limbs were leaden and my thoughts incoherent, exactly as if I were sleep-deprived, drugged, hungover or all three. Did I have the flu? A bug? The dreaded glandular fever? A little unnerved, but thinking I must just need a nap, I closed the book and placed it on the desk, before crawling into the cool bed and under the duvet, back into the space I had vacated only an hour or so previously. I thought after some sleep I would jump up and get cracking, renewed. I thought maybe a coffee and a quick walk around the block might clear my head. I thought many things. But I never once thought that this might be my new state or that living this half-life, as if someone had unplugged me, might be my new 'normal'.

This is something that I have never admitted, but that was the last time during this important period that I opened a book to study.

That afternoon is sharp in my memory. I remember feeling instant relief, pure joy, as I lay my head on the pillow and fell back into a deep and restful sleep.

Mum woke me some hours later.

'You were asleep!' she said, somewhat astonished, having, I am sure, expected to find me reading, writing notes, cramming, keeping pace with the plan on the wall.

'Yep, just nodded off.' I yawned.

'Sorry for waking you, you must be tired, all that revision. Can I get you anything? A drink? Something to eat?'

I shook my head. 'Just going to have twenty minutes.'

'Of course.' She smiled as she backed out of the room and closed my bedroom door.

This was when it began, I suppose, the lying about what was really going on with me and, as important, the sleeping. This desire to sleep arrived coupled with the realisation that the pull of my mattress was far stronger than my desire to achieve my grades.

Sleep. Escape. Oblivion.

These were the things I craved more than a place at any university. More than a fresh start. More than adventure. More than the promised bright future. There was nothing in the whole world I would have chosen over the opportunity to lay my head on that pillow, pull the duvet up and disappear.

I was vaguely aware of the hours passing, of time ticking by. I carried an underlying hum of guilt over the fact that I was not engaged with the work, not revising, which only made my waking hours more uncomfortable. I avoided all the competitive conversations on social media about how much people had revised and what they had studied. I couldn't cope with knowing how many hours they were putting in. They exhausted me and made it feel like I was falling way behind. Breakfast, lunch and supper loosely punctuated the days, and I even managed trips to school for revision sessions and to talk to tutors. In fact, one tutor in particular, Dr P, who had always supported me, now pressed me again and again to hand in the final piece of coursework needed to finish the course and to secure my mark and my future.

'You do know the project needs to be finished, Josh, don't you? You are working on it?'

'Yes,' I lied to her too. And it felt like shit.

I wish I could say I had a plan, that I intended to jump up and crack on, but I didn't. I *couldn't* think – not about the project, not about anything. It was as if I existed in that moment when you first open your eyes in an unfamiliar place, when it takes a second to come to and for any sort of clarity to land. Only it didn't. I didn't come to. I was vacant and vague, distracted and a bit confused. There was no plan. And I didn't have the first clue about how to tell her or anyone else this, not only because I didn't have the confidence, but I didn't have the words. I didn't know what was happening to me.

I remember the look she gave me, holding my eyeline a second or two longer than either of us was comfortable with, as if she suspected I wasn't being truthful, but refusing to believe this of one of her star pupils, the boy to whom she had thrown a rope when he was drowning in insecurity and lack of self-esteem, the boy whose life she had changed with one sentence:

'You have a gift, Josh, you can study this to the highest level if you want to.'

And I did want to, didn't I? This after all was what the last few years had been about; all that work, all the effort, the mental anguish, all were leading to this point when I would get a grade and head off to university to make my dreams come true.

It felt easier to lie to her that I was working than tell her the truth: that I just wanted to close my eyes, lie down and let everything drift overhead.

Study leave was for me leave to sleep. Now, I understand the idea of sleep; that you indulge in it for a solid eight hours or so and wake feeling refreshed and ready to face the day, I get it. I even understand the importance of it at a biological level. The act of sleep itself: vital for muscle repair, memory consolidation and the release of hormones which regulate growth and appetite. But suddenly this was not the case for me and hasn't been since this time. Not once in the past few years have I enjoyed the restorative sleep which I used to take for granted. Yes, I sleep a lot, an awful lot, but the quality of my sleep is poor and despite dedicating hour upon hour to it, I can never have enough. I am never refreshed, always ready to drop off and I want more, more, more . . . Sleep is my drug, my addiction, and the bed my preferred means of getting my hit. I plan my life around naps and longer periods of sleeping, and it often feels that these pillars of sleep are what keep me propped up, as if I am only able to face the world and undertake any chore or activity because I know that the escape of sleep is just around the corner like a reward for any and all actions. Sleep is a powerful master and one to which I am entirely beholden.

According to the journal *CNS Drugs*: 'Fatigue is a frequently reported symptom in major depressive disorder, occurring in over

90 per cent of patients. Clinical presentations of fatigue within major depressive disorder encompass overlapping physical, cognitive and emotional aspects.'[8]

And it was when I was supposed to be studying for the most important exams I was ever going to take that sleep and my need of it took hold. The timing was, as they say, fucking awful.

I continued to stall on the handing in of my Biology project, the final piece of coursework. I became even more evasive about seeing Dr P, avoided communicating with her altogether. She was and is the last person in the world I wanted to let down and yet I did let her down, big time. Even admitting that to you makes me feel a bit sick. I don't know how to apologise to her. I don't know how to explain. But I do know she deserved better.

The project was not beyond me, not at all; I knew what I had to do. I understood it completely, the content and plan were in my head, notes were jotted, research finished and the design formulated. The problem, which felt insurmountable, was getting it down on paper. I was at a loss as to how I ordered the information in my brain into any semblance of a project, even if I could figure out how to stay awake long enough. It was as if each thought had to be dragged through thick, sticky treacle, making every idea sluggish.

Fortunately, my dyslexia had never really held me back in my chosen subject. I found that so much could be passed on with the use of a diagram, a graph and, of course, my terrible, terrible handwriting. But this was not about being dyslexic. This was much bigger than that. It was something different; as though I had lost the connection between my thoughts and how to express them, like someone had cut the wires or a dam had been put up in my mind, an impenetrable wall holding back all ambition and the desire to achieve. And worse still, it took all my energy to power the dam, meaning I constantly felt like I was running on empty and in circles.

I was weak, fatigued and I couldn't wait for it to pass because it was exhausting. I would rest a pen on a blank page or let my fingers hover over the keyboard of the laptop, but it was no good. I could spend hours this way, poised, paralysed and too tired to function. It was like trying to write with soft spaghetti – futile and pointless. I continued to feel wave after wave of tiredness wash over me that no amount of sleep could alleviate. It wasn't just the ordinary ache of muscles and the sore eyes of those in need of rest; this was something deep and dark that I had not experienced before. I would open my eyes and immediately close them again. It was a bone-deep fatigue where I could barely raise a hand, let alone walk, this in conjunction with what I can only describe as a fog, a thought-altering, confusing fug that had permeated my brain, making all logical thought and rational planning impossible. At the same time, it zapped me of all mental energy, which was only mirrored by the physical exhaustion.

It was a downward spiral that I had neither the energy nor inclination to try to climb out of. And it was frightening too. This was my brain we were talking about. I had long since given up hope of my body ever propelling me into an A team and knew that with my dodgy joints and various aches and pains, my physical being was not always reliable. It let me down often, sometimes so much so that getting up and down stairs or in and out of a bath felt like a huge task. But my brain? My brain was a different story. I had always been able to rely on it one hundred per cent. It was all I had.

Clever Josh . . .

Smart Josh . . .

Dr Josh . . .

These and other similar phrases had been shouted in my direction since I had been small, and the thought of my brain failing me, letting me down? What did that leave? It was almost more than I could contemplate. And yet this was precisely what had started to happen.

Mum and Simeon would ferry cups of tea or squash, sandwiches, soup, anything to sustain me while I was, in their belief, locked away, hitting the books. I'd hate the sound of their feet on the stairs, knowing I was going to have to pretend. My door hinge squeaked when it opened and I came to hate that squeak, a forerunner to contact. I hate to think about it even now, long after we have moved. I would look up briefly when they came into the room and even run my finger down a page or type a letter or two on a screen. They would smile at me knowingly, proudly, and leave whatever the offering on the edge of my desk.

Those looks of misplaced pride were like tiny knives that lodged in my chest. As the door closed behind them I would fold in half. Literally fold, either laying my head on my arms on the desk or sinking down into the chair, where I would sit slumped, too tired, too spent to even sit up straight. And always, always with eyelids that were like weighted magnets, drawn down and pulling me deeper, deeper into the dark slumber of escape that my mind and body craved.

It was inevitable, I guess, but no less horrible when Dr P did what she of course had to do and contacted my parents with her concerns. Simeon has told me since that she called him or emailed him.

I am struggling to make Josh understand the importance of this. Where is the final piece of work? Where is his project?

I remember sitting down at the kitchen table with rocks of despair lining my gut, knowing what Mum and Simeon were going to say and not having the first clue about how to answer. I felt blind panic and a sick, sick feeling of failure that left me hollow. I felt fearful and yet strangely vacant. Mum asked if there had been a mix-up.

'Where's the project, Joshy? Where is it?'

And in my head I heard that primary school teacher shouting in my face, 'Why can't you do it, Josh? Everyone else can do it!'

And not for the first time I thought, 'Yeah, why can't you do it, Josh? What the fuck is wrong with you?'

Chapter Seven

Amanda

'Feeling our way in the dark'

'Hope smiles from the threshold of the year to come, whispering "it will be happier" . . .'

Alfred Tennyson

It's fair to say that we were living in a happy bubble until around the time of Josh's study leave before his A levels. Our home dynamic was a lovely one with Simeon around more, thankfully, now that his change of role in the army saw him travelling a little less, and me happily writing book after book after book and popping up on TV screens and radio shows.

It seemed to come out of nowhere, but I noticed a sudden change in Josh's behaviour. He was irritable and tired. Slamming doors. Not answering my questions. Choosing not to shower. Eating dinner quickly and leaving Simeon, Ben and me at the dinner table, as if our company was the last thing he wanted. He was short with me, snappy. Now, don't get me wrong, it wasn't that he used to regularly sit and chew the fat over a cuppa or open up about how he was feeling, and I was certainly not party to all that was going on his life, but this felt different. I would say he had in recent years carried the reticence and slight grumpiness of a typical teenage boy, grunting his one-word replies to even the most wordy of questions and rolling his eyes at everything I did and everything I said. Having grown up with three brothers, I knew this was all quite standard. But this change in him was a marked one from the almost chipper, brighter Josh that had been around since his 'Gabblers' win and the smiley Josh who had ripped open envelopes and beamed at the offers to study. I put it down to the pressure of exams. And I understood.

Ben seemed to be coping well, but Josh not so much. We knew these exams were kind of a big deal, no matter how hard we tried to play it down. I was wary of not adding to his stress, but at the same time really wanted him to do well, to achieve all the things that I (naively) thought might make him happy. Simeon and I discussed it and consulted that well-known parenting tool, Google – where there was no shortage of articles and studies on the terrible effects of exam pressure. I think we read nearly all of them and agreed that the best thing would be to give Josh plenty of space, support him where necessary, help where we were able and do all in our power to coax him over the line where his prize would be his place at university.

Easy peasy.

Much to our joy, he had started to show an interest in going out with his peers, this a fairly new development. The pubs and clubs on The Triangle in Bristol were more often than not their destination, where they queued in a pack with fake IDs clutched in their sweaty palms. I guess it's not conventional parenting, but I took great delight when Josh came home a little sloshed with a lopsided smile, proof that my son was, in the great race towards adulthood, able to relax, socialise, keep pace with his school friends and explore the world, in which I had no doubt he was going to be the most wonderful citizen! We told the boys we were happy they were dipping a toe into this grown-up environment and that as long as they never told us a lie and we always knew where they were, we were good. They promised this would always be the case and I was happy. We believed them. I can't think about those evenings when I opened the front door to Josh at eighteen, leaning on the door frame, often propped up by Ben, without a surge of fond reminiscence. Simeon and I would fall in bed and laugh about our boys, going out and carving their places in the world, boy–men with so many wonderful things lying in wait. My happiness was premature and now more than a little embarrassing.

Because these activities stopped.

All of it stopped.

Suddenly, a little way before his exams, Josh preferred to stay in, declining party invitations from his brother and mates. I must confess I was torn; feeling a little bit delighted that he was so keen to stay in and study, his drive and dedication to achieve his goal were something I greatly admired, and yet at the same time I was concerned that he wasn't letting his hair down and taking time out to relax. As nearly every article we read on the subject suggested, the key to successful student life during exam time was balance, and it didn't appear that Josh had any. It was all work and no play, or so I thought.

It was hard to get him up in the morning to go to school for study sessions and he was keen to go back to bed the second he arrived home. I found this irritating, unable to understand how he was happy to spend so much of his time horizontally with the curtains drawn, especially while Ben was out running, socialising or chatting to us downstairs. There it was again, that mirror to Josh's life, grossly unfair on both of the boys and yet almost impossible not to look at. All attempts at conversation drew a blank.

'Are you okay, Joshy?'

'Yep.'

'Do you need any help with anything?'

'Nope.'

'Are you worried about anything?'

'Nope.'

'You know you can talk to us about anything, anytime?'

. . . Eye roll, accompanied by heavy sigh.

With the exams drawing nearer, Simeon came home one evening with skin that looked ashen, his expression fraught.

'What's the matter?' My thoughts raced, trying to figure out what might have happened at work and my first thought was that he had been told he was going away on tour again, something I live in dread of, but no. This time, his worry was not centred on a hot place far away, but was somewhere a lot, lot closer to home.

'I received a call from Dr P . . .' he began.

I remember laughing, nervous laughter no doubt, as Simeon explained that Josh had failed to hand in his final piece of work and that without it, his predicted A* would now not be possible – how could it when the project constituted a big chunk of the overall marks?

'Well, that can't be right! They must have made a mistake . . . Have they lost it?' My question was as ridiculous as it sounds, but at the time felt like the most logical thing to ask. It was to me far more likely that this vital project had been mislaid, that it was someone else's fault, rather than the unpalatable thought that Josh might be self-sabotaging his efforts. I could not conceive how it might be possible that he could fall at the final hurdle, not after everything he had been through.

It made no sense to me, none at all.

I was thoroughly confused and conflicted. I had prided myself on being one of those parents who could say with confidence, 'I don't mind what my children do, what path they take, as long as they are happy.'

And I thought I meant it. And yet the idea that Josh might be throwing away his chance, with me believing that happiness lay at the end of this academic path . . . I felt sick at the prospect. I also thought I knew what was going on with my kids, repeatedly telling them that they could talk to us about anything, anything at all.

We hastily arranged to go and see Josh's head of year, let's call him Mr G, who was kind, patient and smart. He calmly explained there was a danger that unless Josh really, really applied himself, tried to catch up, worked hard and concentrated particularly on handing in the required project, the rough deadlines for which had already passed, he would be staring at a huge mountain of work, and quite simply there would be too little time left to climb the mountain, meaning he could only fail. It was the only option. Failure. Simeon and I thanked him and left his office to drive home in silence. We were a little bit numb and a whole lot lost for words.

'What should we do, Simeon?' I whispered as he pulled the car into the driveway. We sat there staring at the house, as if neither of us particularly wanted to go in.

'I don't know,' came his honest reply. This was not what I wanted to hear, but it was the truth: we were stumped.

I went into Josh's room and sat on the end of his bed, nudging him awake. The room smelled sour; I wanted to fling open the windows and rip off his bed linen before shoving it on a long, hot wash, but I was aware that this felt a lot like his nest, his refuge and was wary of disturbing him in the one place he clearly felt comfortable. It was amazing how quickly this state of affairs had become normal. Josh had in the last few weeks taken to his bed and stayed there. If I suggested that he got up or asked how the studying was going he looked nothing short of tortured. Ben, I noticed, kept his distance and this I understood; he had his own exam pressure to deal with, his own less complicated life to live. Simeon and I agreed that normal behaviour would no doubt resume after the exams and frankly we couldn't wait. But this call from Dr P was, for us at least, a wake-up call. Was there something more going on with Josh?

I concentrated on keeping my voice calm and encouraging, wanting to make it clear that I was there to help him, not scold him.

'Darling, I am so worried about you. You need to finish your project; Dr P has been in touch and we've been to see Mr G, who was lovely about the whole thing, but he's worried about you too, we all are. How can we help you? What can we do, Josh?'

'You can leave me alone and let me sleep,' came his grumbled reply and he turned over, pulling the duvet up over his head.

I remember feeling utterly bewildered. What was the right course of action? If I got mad would he produce the work? Probably not, in fact it might make him withdraw even more. Should we bribe, coax, encourage or shout . . . all felt futile. We were after all talking about an eighteen-year-old, an adult technically with the knowledge in his head and a will of his own, how could we *make* him do anything? Plus, we were not the kind of parents who used harsh discipline, instead seeing childrearing as a gentle, ongoing thing that required steering constantly and not the sudden flare of anger, shouting or laying down of the rules when things went wrong. And, anyway, things had never really gone wrong before.

Simeon and I were at a loss as to how to handle the situation. It was a horrible and frightening realisation that we just didn't know how best to advise Josh. And this made us question how we parented; we were the grown-ups and we were supposed to know the answers. We put faith, as we always did, in talking things through and calmly trying to figure out the best course of action. I probably cried as well, just for good measure. (Yes, Josh – I have read your views on my constant tears!) There was an order of events in which things needed addressing and we figured the best thing to do was get the damned project finished as a matter of urgency. Hindsight is, of course, a wonderful thing. It was like we couldn't see the real problem, looking at one of the symptoms (Josh not working) and trying to fix that rather than taking a helicopter view and asking *why* he wasn't working. It felt like there was the most enormous time pressure.

Josh has to get this project done and he is running out of time!

He has to hand his project in or everything is in jeopardy!

We are letting Dr P and Mr G down after all they have done for us!

I can only imagine how it must have seemed to Josh. I can now see that what we *should* have done was say, 'Don't think about the project! Forget it! Nothing matters, darling, nothing!' and simply wrapped him up and held him tight and told him the only thing to concentrate on was feeling better and getting back on his feet. But at this point we didn't know he was ill and thought it was a blip, a protest, a reaction, whatever. I guess I had been conditioned and thought these stupid exams were important. I still believed they were his ticket and I was overly concerned with him giving it up. As I sit here writing, shame laces these memories along with a huge jab of regret. It is fair to say that my decisions were based on two things: ignorance of what might be best for my son's mental health, and my desires for Josh, driven partly by what I thought was best for his future – my own standard – and all propped up by my belief that the golden life at university might be just like it was in the movies. I thought that he would go, excel, graduate, fall in love and throw his mortar board hat in the air for the final photograph.

The End.

I'm sorry, Josh.

I am so, so sorry.

Simeon, as ever when called upon, leapt into action, helping Josh as much as he was able with the project, sitting beside him at the table while Josh stared blankly at a computer screen, looking away occasionally to yawn or run his fingers through his hair. It was as if he wasn't present and it took me back to when he was a small

81

child and had to write an essay, the slow, drawn-out, torturous process of trying to get him to engage and having to spell and re-spell every single syllable while he peppered the page with random dots and dashes, thinking this constituted punctuation. I sat on the sidelines, hollering words of encouragement, making endless cups of tea and tiptoeing around the thoughts of what might happen if Josh didn't wake up and shape up. The tension was palpable and Ben took to his room too, not to sleep but I think to avoid the atmosphere, and who could blame him?

Simeon and I discussed the matter in private, often before we fell asleep. We felt the stress as a couple, chatting back and forth about the situation in which we as a family found ourselves.

What's wrong with him?

Could it be glandular fever?

Is he on drugs?

Might he be gay and struggling with his sexuality?

Has something happened that he can't talk about, a trauma?

Answers were in short supply and we felt then, pretty much as we do now, all these years later, like we were trying to feel our way in the dark; one wrong move and we were all doomed. I am beyond thankful for being able to take Simeon's hand in the darkness. It gives me strength. It keeps me going . . .

The simple truth: this was the start of it.

We were poised on a crumbling cliff edge and the whole she-bang was about to fall. We just didn't know it.

Chapter Eight

JOSH

'THERAPY. *TICK!*'

'I am in that temper that if I were under water I would
scarcely kick to come to the top.'

John Keats

I cobbled together a project of sorts. I don't really remember what
or how, but it was certainly not the one I had envisaged or planned,
nor was it, I knew, of the quality to gain the grade I had previously
achieved, not even close; it was a poor substitution, but at least it
was something. Very little pride was taken in it. But then it's hard
to take pride in much that is executed while in a state of utter
exhaustion. I just wanted it done and out of the way, in truth,
more concerned with making the uncomfortable questioning over
it stop than the end result. It was all more than I could handle.
Handing it in brought some small sense of relief, but little else.
Dr P was understandably frosty, she must have felt so let down,
so disappointed, and I cringe to look back and think about it, but

at the time, even this had little effect on me. The numbness had started to set in.

So I handed in the project and I went back to sleep.

There was great debate, both between my parents and between my parents and teachers, as to whether I should, or indeed would be able to sit the final exams. I felt indifferent, as if they were talking about someone else, and clearly this was part of the problem. The question was whether it would be better to sit them and try to get a grade, any grade, or whether it was better for my mental health not to sit them and swallow the big fat zero. I was quite happy to be guided and take the advice offered: that being, we would see how I felt on the day. It felt like the best compromise but was in reality the biggest cop-out. I know now I should have said I'm not doing them and someone should have agreed. I say that without blame or judgement, fully aware that everyone was doing their best with no experience or plan, but when your brain is so fogged that you can't decide whether to turn left or right and even choosing between coffee or tea feels like too much of a decision, it really helps for someone to take the reins and guide you.

Mum tentatively suggested it might be an idea for me to go and speak to someone, an expert, a therapist or a counsellor, whoever might help. She tried to make the suggestion sound casual, but I could tell by her manner, her hesitancy, this felt a bit like starting along a path that she did not particularly want me to walk, and possibly one she did not want to walk either, and I understood. It was a big deal: the start of a dialogue where words like mental health, depression, breakdown and all other unpalatable ailments when talking about your child would start to pepper our language. It made it real, for her at least. Too numb to really care or participate in that dialogue, it was already very real to me.

With a long NHS waiting list, too long to be seen pre-exams, she found a private therapist who dealt specifically with exam stress and anxiety, and who might, she thought, be able to give me some tips on how to get through this tricky time. I could see through her smile, the one designed to convince me and everyone else that everything was going to be fine. If anything, her mask irritated me. I didn't know what was happening, but I knew things were far from fine and at some level I just wanted her to acknowledge that and then maybe I would not have to pretend too.

The appointment was made in hushed tones, like it was a shameful thing, and one day after school she took me to the clinic on the outskirts of Bristol. As we drove up the winding drive to the once grand house, now hospital, I could tell she was nervous, repeating that I shouldn't be worried and giving me the most basic advice as if I were a child.

'Be sure to tell them how you feel, Joshy. Don't be embarrassed or worried, there is nothing you can say that they haven't heard a million times before . . . I mean, sometimes people struggle with things like their nerves or sexuality and . . .'

'I'm not gay, Mum, and if I was, I know it wouldn't be a problem, of course not.'

This much I did know.

'Of course not,' she echoed. 'I am just trying to think of all the reasons why you might feel a little out of sorts, about anything that might be on your mind . . .' She let this trail.

I felt a bit sorry for her then and could see that she, like me, wished it were as simple as identifying what the problem was, highlighting one thing that we could all try to understand, because then we could go about trying to figure out how to fix it.

I waited outside the therapist's room on a squeaky red leather couch and filled in a form attached to a clipboard – easier than it sounds, as I only had to put ticks by the appropriate responses.

Are you happy or sad?
Sad. Tick.
Do you take regular medication?
No. Tick.

Does your mood affect your daily life?

Yes. Tick.

Have you ever considered suicide?

No. Tick.

And at that moment in time, this was the truth.

To be honest the therapist was disappointing; we did not connect at all and he was not someone I would ever have chosen to confide in. He didn't seem smart, avoided eye contact and was, if anything, a little nervous, relying more than I would have thought on the crappy form I had filled in with ticks than anything else, and all whilst sitting in a therapist pose with his legs crossed and his fingers occasionally stroking his chin in contemplation. I had kind of hoped he would be brilliant, take one look at me and give me the answer – ta-dah! – like a magician revealing his trick. Because it might have been early days in terms of my journey into depression but I already wanted out. Sadly, this was not the case. His questions were predictable and slow in coming, his answers to my questions were standard, until eventually he asked if I could think of *'one trauma that might be making me feel low or causing my anxiety? Something that had maybe occurred in the past? Anything? Anything at all?'*

I shook my head. There was nothing. He looked disappointed and more than a little stumped. I understood this too. It was like going back to the conversation in the car with my mum. It would have been so much easier if there *had* been one thing that had cracked the surface of my happiness, one thing that I could detail, an event or happening on to which my anxiety and general malaise might be pinned. At least then we would all know what we were dealing with and no doubt the rubbish therapist would have a chart to consult that might, if nothing else, take the discussion forward. Although I suspect his chart would look a bit like:

If the answer is yes – offer medication.

If the answer is no – offer medication.

He offered me medication.

I politely refused and got back in the car. I was aware of how medication altered your brain chemistry and that was not a route I wanted to take – no thank you. My brain was clearly altered enough right now. Mum looked at me, her smile had been replaced with an expression of hope. This I think partly because she wanted answers. Didn't we all, Mandy! And also because I know the appointment had cost a decent sum when money was tight and I suspect she hoped at some level that it had not been wasted.

'Did you like talking to him?'

No. Tick.

'Was it useful, Joshy?'

No. Tick.

'Do you think you might get some benefit from going again?'

No. Tick.

And to think we had paid a hefty fee for the privilege.

We drove home in silence and I felt a new layer of rocks in my gut, this time they were made up of guilt. *I am causing Mum and Simeon worry. I am letting them down . . .*

'It'll all be okay, Joshy.' She patted my arm. I did not believe her. But it felt easier to say nothing.

I went back to bed and, leaving it almost up until the day to decide, I sat the exams. Mum and Simeon had said I might as well, seeing as I was going to get zero if I didn't turn up, what did I have to lose? This sounded logical and I agreed, but on the day itself there was nothing logical about my thought process. I wanted to cry. I did cry, I think.

I trudged into school with a headache that felt like my skull was splitting, a gut that churned with nerves and a once decent brain that had been replaced with scrambled egg. I felt strangely removed from the situation, a bit like I was watching myself from afar. I kept looking at the big clock on the wall of the gym, not for the same reason as the other candidates who pushed their pens across the paper with lightning speed with one eye on the time, but so I could work out how soon this would be over and how quickly I could crawl back into the warm, dark space beneath my duvet.

This was I think when the hazy confusion started to set in.

My memory was not so sharp, time felt skewed and still the pull of my bed was irresistible and being in it the best thing I could imagine. I overate, and not just overate, I ate rubbish and gained weight, this did little for my already fragile self-esteem. Now, I didn't like the way my mind worked, I didn't like all the things I could not do due to my crappy joint problem and I didn't like the way I looked. A hat-trick.

I had started to unravel.

My self-imposed exile and social exclusion came to an end, largely due to the fact that my desire to drink and seek escape through alcohol was greater than my desire for solitude and so I left the house on the odd occasion to drink. Heavily. There was a certain kudos in being able to drink more than my peers and when indulging, I necked booze at breakneck speed to self-medicate. I think it's fair to say I felt something – maybe a small flush of status at how impressed they were with my drinking ability. It's a strange dichotomy that whilst drinking to the cheers in the pub, I simultaneously felt nothing, further numbed by the alcohol and able for a short time to escape even more from the world. There aren't many worse feelings than being lonely in a crowded room. We have never lived in a more connected world, yet loneliness is only increasing. We as a society must look at the value of these connections; a thousand Instagram followers aren't worth as much as one person who you can communicate honestly and openly with, at least in my opinion.

Looking back, I can see that this period of time around my exams was when I experienced my first depressive episode. Sadly, it was not the last and in comparison to how low I would eventually sink, this was a fucking cakewalk.

Photographs

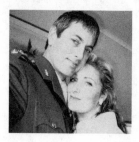

So I married my soldier. This was taken on our wedding day, which was just the two of us, no flowers, no fancy frock, no reception. We came home afterwards and had a pizza out of the freezer and a cup of tea. The next day, Simeon went on tour in Iraq.

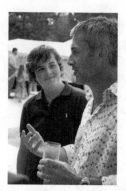

Mandy: Josh aged twelve with Simeon. I love the way he is looking at him.

Josh: We were at a summer party and it was a good day. Simeon was on good form and I felt proud of our family.

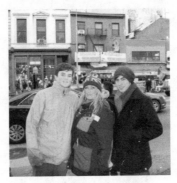

Mandy: Josh, Ben and me on our first family trip to New York. It was Christmas. Boys were aged thirteen. It was so very cold but that didn't dampen the holiday spirit! We were all a little bit in awe of this city we had only seen before in the movies!

Josh: Shortly after this photograph was taken, I high-fived a hanging strobe light and the electric shock threw me off my feet! I laugh every time I see it and think, why did I do that?

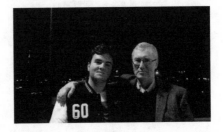

Mandy: Josh with his grandad in his first few weeks at Southampton University. We went to take him out for supper. The look on my dad's face says it all – how proud we all were of our boy . . . I can't stand Josh's expression, a slight smile, but his eyes tell a different story . . .

Josh: I remember this night. My parents and grandparents came to take me out for supper. I could tell they wanted to see me doing well and were beaming at me. I told them everything was okay. But it wasn't, not at all. I remember being glad to wave them goodbye.

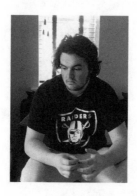

Josh at home. He had gained weight and was either lethargic or angry. It was like walking on eggshells around him and it was hard to fathom why, because as far as we were concerned he had this great life! Little did we know what was around the corner . . .

Josh: I hate to look at this photograph. I was in turmoil and was desperate to be alone, even though I was lonely when I was alone. But then I was also lonely in a crowd. It was the start of the very darkest period for me and if I could go back to then I know I would need to ask for help sooner. Talk it through.

Chapter Nine

Amanda

'Have you ever been to Aberdeen?'

'Life is not meant to be easy, my child; but take courage: it can be delightful.'

George Bernard Shaw

Josh's A level results came in early one August morning. It was a day that had loomed large, red-ringed on the calendar, and one I had done my very best to ignore. It was like waiting for the results of a health check and that phrase that is nearly always offered as a sticking plaster – 'No point worrying until you know you have something to worry about . . .' So easy to say and actually it does nothing for your worried state, apart from make you feel guilty for worrying, as if it is a weakness rather than a human reaction. It was *partly* true in that as long as the results weren't in, there was still a chance that Josh had somehow done the impossible in that exam hall and would get the required grades, take his place at St Andrews and his life would get back on track . . . And I guess by default, so could mine. We could then, as a family, put this summer of stomach-churning concern over his brain fog, his apathy and his sleepy-headed lack of interaction behind us. Oh my God! My ignorance, naivety and lack of understanding were breathtaking, but no less damaging for that. I had repeated the mantra 'it'll all be okay!' so often to anyone who asked, my parents and wider family included, that I think I had started to believe it.

'How's Josh doing?'

'Oh, he'll be fine! It'll all be okay!'

Josh had said very little about the exams once they were over; he had in fact said very little about anything and had spent the summer either drinking with a select group of friends, attending the odd music festival or, of course, indulging in his favourite pastime: sleeping. I can't pretend that there weren't times when his slumbering body caused me great irritation. No less so than when Simeon and I were running around like the proverbial blue-arsed flies trying to work and keep the house running while he lay in his room, seemingly oblivious. It took all of my strength not to yell:

'Why don't you get up?'

'Did you not hear the doorbell? We missed a delivery!'

'Why don't you have a bath or go for a walk?'

'Would it hurt you to bring your dirty cups and plates downstairs?'

'Why am I having to collect your laundry? It's not fair, Josh!'

'Enough already! Snap out of it! Just snap out of it!'

I wish I could go back and do it differently. I wish a lot of things.

This day, results day, was one that will stay with me always.

Josh was, unusually, out of bed before midday. He had opened the email with his final results in it, alone. Ben had done the same before going out to meet up with his mates. Simeon and I sat with Josh at the kitchen table with the French doors open and a warm breeze flowing in. The sun was shining and birds were singing. It would have been a perfect day were it not for the email that had arrived on Josh's laptop earlier. That and you could have cut the atmosphere with a knife, the air heavy with expectation and dread.

The chatter among our social networks and in WhatsApp groups was of course full of the successes of Josh's peers, and I certainly didn't begrudge them that. I know the relief and joy those students and their families must have felt at knowing that was it, job done, whilst popping corks and planning accommodation and travel for all the new adventures that lay ahead. But I'd be lying if I didn't say it made a tough day even tougher.

We were not cracking open a bottle or packing a suitcase; instead we sat with fingers coiled into palms, hearts racing and words of solace stuttering on our nervous tongues. Simeon and I were actually over the moon that Josh had, *surprisingly*, incredibly and brilliantly managed to pass all three subjects with no more than his residual learning and not a scrap of revision – quite amazing. I was proud! Genuinely so. But Josh's face told me there was no point in plying him with platitudes when his dreams of attending St Andrews lay in tatters. He had not achieved the result they had asked for and upon which his place was dependent, and had *unsurprisingly* dropped a couple of grades, gaining an A, B and D. God, I have just read that sentence again and I can't believe how inconsequential and ridiculous it feels to have written it. Three little letters A, B and D – three letters that had such power and which felt so very significant. Three grades that most people would be overjoyed with! How utterly, utterly ridiculous it all is. What a bloody stupid way of measuring smartness – but that, my friend, is a whole other conversation for a whole other day. His grades, acquired without scribe or assistance, were indeed fantastic, in the upper region of grades attained nationally, but of course for Josh they were a significant drop, a marker of how far he had fallen mentally – and crucially not enough for him to take up his place at the university of his choice.

'They . . . they won't let me go. I . . . I didn't do enough,' he managed, face pale and eyes misting.

'You did great, darling, against all the odds, you did really great!' we tried, but he just stared at us, his gaze calling us liars.

Simeon galvanised us and pulled the telephone on to the kitchen table and opened his laptop. 'Right, we are going to go through clearing.' This is the system where universities advertise spaces now available and students log in if their grades were worse or better than expected to try and enrol on a course. It felt a bit like a virtual game of musical chairs, with students who had failed to make their grades snapping up an ever-decreasing number of places. 'Don't worry, Josh! It will all be okay.' There it was, that 'go to' phrase again, no longer truly convincing anyone.

Having logged into the Universities and Colleges Admission Service site we began to trawl through lists, looking for universities where they had places on offer to study Biology. I knew for a fact there was a spot going in St Andrews, one of the most prestigious places to study in the UK and located north of Edinburgh in Scotland, and took some small measure of comfort from the thought of a young person like Josh, who had maybe achieved better grades than they had expected, calling up and being given the wonderful news. Looking back, it was farcical really, as if Simeon and I were taking part in the crappiest pantomime, throwing out positive lines wherever possible to fill the deafening silence.

'Ooh Nottingham! Lovely, let's try there! Hull? Wow! Hull is brilliant!'

My face ached from all the false smiling while Josh stared at his lap. Had I arrived on the scene without any emotional involvement, a stranger, I would have taken one look at the boy and listened to Simeon's frantic list-making, amid my chatter of positive suggestion and I would have called a halt, citing that it was all too much, too fast . . . *Let the boy breathe . . . not everyone has to go to unibloodyversity . . .*

But I can only say that hindsight is a wonderful thing. I had sworn when he was born to always fight for him and this was me doing just that with Simeon by my side, fighting for Josh's place.

I shan't ever forget the sight of my son sitting with the phone in his shaking palms, dialling the numbers, taking deep breaths and closing his eyes as he spoke with a quaver to his voice, barely able to get the words out and crying, as he was put on hold while Simeon and I cried with him.

'Hello, my . . . my name is Josh. I have just got my results and was wondering if you had any places to study Biology . . .'

We dictated what we thought it best for him to say and he scrawled the script on a tatty piece of paper, which I carry with me to this day. It reminds me of that terrible morning and teaches me to look beyond the moment: to try to be the stranger who can see more than what is immediately obvious and to maybe ask different questions. On that day, instead of rushing to help Josh with a script and putting the phone in his hands, I would *not* now say, 'How do you fancy going to Swansea?' but would ask, 'Is this what you want? Do you think university is right for you right now? If at all?'

Finally, after several flat-out 'no's, there was a ray of hope when Aberdeen University offered him a place. If I could, I would have jumped down the telephone line and kissed the woman on the other end of the phone. She had thrown him a lifeline. I knew he might not accept a place at Aberdeen, a place he knew very little about and where he knew no one, but that was not the point: someone had wanted him and when you felt as unwanted and as lost as Josh did on that day, it meant the world.

'Oh, Josh! Aberdeen! How wonderful! Aberdeen!' I enthused. 'That will be lovely! Aberdeen! I think it's on the coast. You love the sea, you can go sailing! I think there's lots of fish and hillwalking.'

'Hillwalking?' Simeon asked quizzically, subtly pointing out that Josh had never hill-walked in his life.

'Have you ever been to Aberdeen, Mum?' Josh asked quietly.

'No. No I haven't,' I had to admit.

'Do you know exactly where it is?'

'Erm, no, no I don't, not exactly . . .'

I think we all laughed for the first and last time that day. And in truth if it had been what Josh had wanted then we of course would have supported his decision to study there. It was only when I looked at it on a map and saw that it was nearly a nine-hour drive door to door or a very expensive, non-direct flight that I felt some misgivings. My overriding thought being that if Josh needed our help or support, it would be impossible to get to him quickly. Finally, an offer came from the University of Southampton, which was only a couple of hours away by car from our home. Simeon and I were hugely relieved. Josh seemed a little removed from the whole process, his gaze off-centre.

I can't think about it without tears gathering at the back of my throat and a deep throb of sadness in my chest. It was one of the first times that I had witnessed Josh in a state of anxiety-ridden panic. It was torturous and I felt helpless to intervene and ill-equipped to know what to say and what to do. I hated this day more than most others. I still dream about it. And that's an odd one for me, as there have been days along Josh's journey which were far, far worse in terms of emotional or physical upheaval and yet this day sticks with me and I have tried to figure out why.

The reasons are not easy ones for me to consider, as it is clear that it's much more about me than Josh and forces me to face some unpalatable truths. These being that I fought to keep Josh at a school that I believed would be best for a boy with his dyslexic challenges, ploughing money I could often ill afford into a system I hoped would make him the best version of himself. I think I saw his good results as proof that my monthly pay check deposited into the school's bank account in lieu of a reliable car, holidays, clothes and even trips to the hairdressers had all been worth it. Justification, if you like, for all I had gone without, especially in the early years. I also wanted at some level to demonstrate my son's success to those boys who had excluded or been mean to Josh, and their loud, loud parents. I wanted to show them all that he was not only in the race, but he was winning! I don't feel proud of these feelings, not at all.

Being offered a place to study was wonderful but it was also tempered by the realisation that we still had a long, long way to go to get Josh ready for university, and only a very short time in which to do it. Again, we were back to panicking over a ridiculous and unachievable timescale. Simeon and I were still running blindly, arms out, eyes closed. The only difference was this time in our ignorance, we were fuelled by excitement rather than fear.

Josh responded immediately to the offer from Southampton, as was the protocol, making sure his place was secured, but he did so with no more than a cursory nod. I had expected something more – if not cartwheels of joy then at the very least, relief. It was almost with reluctance that he opened the 'Congratulations' cards sent to him from friends and family before tossing them to one side and going straight back to bed. I think this was the first time I questioned whether he was, as we had believed up until this point, going through something that would end, meaning there would be a day when the sun came out again, restoring him back to the Josh we knew and loved. I missed the boy who had such a capacity for sharp, insightful witticism, but I had to wonder if there was something else at play, something that actually inhibited his ability to feel joy and to have fun. I decided to read about depression, a thought that had nagged at me for a little while now. I let my eyes run down the list of symptoms as listed on www.samaritans.org

Lacking energy or feeling tired

Feeling exhausted all the time

Experiencing 'brain fog', finding it hard to think clearly

Finding it hard to concentrate

Feeling restless and agitated

Feeling tearful, wanting to cry all the time

Not wanting to talk to or be with people

Not wanting to do things you usually enjoy

Using alcohol or drugs to cope with feelings

Finding it hard to cope with everyday things and tasks

Experiencing 'burn out'

I had hoped that this first foray into the world of mental illness would prove my concerns unfounded and thought I might laugh with relief at how wide of the mark my suspicions were, but instead this list sent a shiver along my limbs. My son had, or was showing signs of, nearly all of the above. This was a marker and the first time that I used the word depression. It is a word I have come to detest. A word I dream about and which hovers around the edge of my consciousness no matter what I am doing, who I am with or where I am. A word the misuse of which makes my hackles rise and my gut jump.

DEPRESSION.

I said it out loud and it felt like a weight, a sharp rock lodged in my throat, which affected my speech and my breathing and quite frankly, it hurt.

I considered the word, which for me conjured images of failure, of bow-headed, broken, bed-bound beings with swollen eyes red-ringed with tears and a pale, haunting apathy that painted them in sadness. I was wary of applying another label to Josh who had been stickered thus his whole life, but deep down I *wanted* him to tell me he felt he might have depression because at least then I would have a word, a phrase, a condition, which might explain, or at least help in the understanding of his symptoms and behaviours. My thought process was that if he could look me in the eye and tell me he was depressed, I could then look others in the eye and tell them my son was depressed and it *would, might, hopefully* put an end to the wishy-washy, vague mumblings of how he was feeling a little 'under the weather', a phrase I had shamefully used both to family and friends. Good God! What the hell does it mean anyway?

Under the weather?

I am irritated by the mere writing of it and can only imagine how it must have felt, as a sufferer of depression, to hear it. Can you imagine living with a long-term illness that erodes all that makes you you and someone describing you as 'a bit under the weather'?

Again, oh, again, again . . . I'm sorry, Josh.

This is yet another example of how my bumbling ineptitude, trying to paint on a smile and make everything good without the first clue of what my boy was going through, might just have made things a whole heap worse.

This label might be useful, appropriate even, a signpost for Josh and all those around him, but at the same time and in equal measure *I did not want* this word nailed to the mast of the ship in which my son sailed.

It's a shameful thing for me to admit, but I did not want that for him, didn't want him to be a person like that – the irony being, of course, HE ALREADY WAS A PERSON LIKE THAT!

And the simple truth is that at some level I didn't want him to tell me he had depression because I honestly did not know what I would do with that information. And instantly we were back to the impossible questions:

How do we treat that?

Where's the cure?

Are there tablets?

Is there a specific doctor you can go and see?

A retreat where you get to sit in the sun and come back fixed?

Would a brisk walk help?

Some homemade soup?

A hug?

I know, I know: ridiculous, all of it ridiculous. With hindsight, I can tell you that it really wasn't that complicated. Deep down I knew that with an admission of this kind from Josh, when and if it was forthcoming, and with the word DEPRESSION painted brightly on the front of the banner behind which we marched, walked and sometimes crawled, our journey was about to begin and I had no idea of the route we should take, what to pack or even where we were heading.

In the weeks before Josh left home for university and Ben started college, the difference in the mental health of my sons was never more apparent. We would whisper to Ben on the landing, telling him that Josh was not well, whilst encouraging him to go out and enjoy himself, waving him off for a night out, before returning to watch Josh sleep. The hope was that if he slept long enough and deep enough he might reach a 'refreshed' state, might wake up with a big overhead stretch, a yawn and a spring in his step – hallelujah! Something which, of course, we now know is impossible to achieve with depression when even getting out of bed, showering or brushing your hair can prove too hard. But nevertheless we watched and hoped, feeding him nutritious meals and reading aloud to him snippets from the prospectus about all the wonderful things the University of Southampton had to offer – 'Ooh, look, Josh, a cinema!' – hoping, I think, that our enthusiasm for the cafes and bars, clubs and societies that ranged from snowboarding to photography might enthuse him a little. They didn't seem to and if anything, I would describe his mood as resigned. He was quiet. Simeon and I discussed it endlessly and we thought that when he arrived on campus and was in the thick of it, student life would absorb him and hopefully ignite the spark we so dearly missed.

It was late on a cold, crisp Sunday morning when Josh crept down the stairs and sat at the kitchen table. He looked grim, unwashed, a little vacant and was still in his pyjamas and dressing gown. Only the day before we had started to gather the things he

101

might need for university – new duvet, pens, plates, cutlery . . . It was like I could hear the clock ticking, counting down until the day he left, and this was the state of him. I didn't know what to do but felt the swell of panic nonetheless. I knew I needed to do *something*. I was making brunch for the family. Simeon was pottering in the garden and Ben was in bed watching TV. It felt somehow easier to talk while I was preoccupied and we were alone.

'So, Joshy, I was thinking about people I have known who've had depression, and I'm not saying you *have*' – wary as ever of putting words in his mouth and of giving him a platform on which to jump that might not have been accurate or helpful – 'and I think that a lot of things they have said or mentioned and their behaviours, well, they seem a lot like the things you have said, or mentioned, and the way you behave . . .'

He looked at me with the same open expression he has had since he was a newborn, the same questioning eyes that stared up at me on his very first day as he rested on my legs when sleep proved evasive, and said, 'Really, Mum? Ya think?'

A different day and a different topic and I would have been laughing: '*I know, right! It looks like a banana, smells like a banana, tastes like a banana, chances are . . .*'

But this was not the time for laughter; this was Josh's brain we were discussing. His beautiful, brilliant, unique, enigmatic and charismatic brain and we were essentially saying that it was a little broken.

'So, are you saying you think you *might* have depression, Josh?' I pushed slowly, in an almost sing-song manner, again trying to defuse the verbal cluster bombs my mouth launched and fired directly at him. With my back to him, tending to a pan on the stove as I made scrambled eggs, I held my breath waiting for him to respond, waiting for a rebuttal, a scathing, comical, insightful retort that might defuse the next explosive in the way only Josh could . . . but he said nothing. And so I turned to the table, smile fixed and . . . and my son was crying. My grown-up boy sat with fat tears running down his face. And he cried like a child, a child who was hurt.

'I'm tired, Mum,' he managed from a mouth contorted with sadness. 'I am so tired.'

Abandoning the stove, I looked at him as my distress matched his own. He was bow-headed and broken, with swollen eyes red-ringed with tears and a pale, haunting apathy that painted him in sadness.

And there it was, the label.

The end and the beginning. We had used the word.

Depression. Josh was suffering with depression.

It was a word that I had heard a lot but had very little under-standing of. Wasn't it just a catch-all for people feeling a little off colour? I remember thinking that if you used the word depression it didn't feel like healing would be quick, recalling how people spoke of 'living with depression' and 'battling depression' rather than 'I once had depression'. This was a blow. Ridiculously, I was still hoping at some level that he would recover the spring in his step and bound off to uni. I remember looking over his shoulder as I held him in my arms while he cried. I could see Simeon in the garden and knew that I was going to wipe out his hopes of an early recovery for Josh when I recounted this moment to him later. I didn't relish it.

I asked softly, 'Do you still think you want to go to uni?'

'Yes.'

'Are you sure? Because—'

'Yes!' He cut me off.

'Do you want to go and talk to someone, Josh? A doctor?'

'No!' he barked.

'They might be able to give you something or maybe they might have advice?'

'No!' he barked again and pushed me away.

I remember watching him jump from the table and run up the stairs and thinking, well, what the hell do we do now?

Chapter Ten

Josh

'A Fresh Start'

'Our whole being is nothing but a fight against the
dark forces within ourselves.'

Henrik Ibsen

The period between leaving school and waiting for the results of
my exams to come out felt like an eternity; it was in fact no more
than eight weeks. Life was on hold and that actually suited me.
Unsurprisingly I slept, slipping deeper and deeper into a state of
melancholy and wanting nothing but isolation. Then strangely,
after results day, which was an emotional one especially for Mum
who went into 'pretend happy' overdrive, which was fucking horrific, it went from feeling like everything was happening in slow
motion to feeling as if life was hurtling at lightning speed, certainly
faster than I could keep steady or upright. I was offered a place at
the University of Southampton – coincidentally where one of my
best friends from school was heading. A university in the Russell

Group with a good reputation for Biology, I should have been chuffed, right? And I was to a degree, but the fist pump of satisfaction offered by my peers at the prospect of going away from home for the first time? Nah, it was nothing like that. The disappointment at not getting to take my place at St Andrews outweighed the relief of the offer from Southampton. The whole thing felt like a failure, like second best. I didn't know it, but my capacity for joy had already been clipped. I reckon my offer could have come via an announcement from the Foo Fighters on the main stage at Glastonbury and been followed up with a drive home in a McLaren P1 and I would have felt the same: a bit meh, almost indifferent. Obviously, looking back I can see that it was a big clue as to my state of mind.

There didn't seem to be much time between accepting the offer and actually moving to Southampton at the beginning of term: just a few weeks, in fact, after sitting at the kitchen table and going through the 'clearing' system to find a place. As I had spent more than the last few weeks in a kind of stupor, I began to quietly panic. I felt apprehensive and wary at the prospect of meeting new people and living in a strange place. The thought of attending lectures and what the academic work might be like didn't enter my head. It felt impossible to imagine. Everyone from family to friends and even others I was yet to meet in person who chatted online, people who were on my course, kept telling me how great it was going to be and how lucky I was to have secured a place. I felt I had no choice but to go with the flow. But it didn't feel great and I didn't feel very lucky. In fact, I felt nothing like the bubbling excitement I had at one time anticipated, but something a lot closer to dread. I was fearful but couldn't accurately pinpoint what I was afraid of. It felt easier to stay quiet.

I was banking on the fact that a new start in a new place might help me shake off the feelings of exhaustion and the sadness that plagued me. I also hoped my inability to focus and study that had messed up my A levels might have passed by the time I moved into the halls of residence, but deep down, and something I never let on, I doubted it. I didn't talk to any of my friends about how I was feeling, didn't mention it to anyone. It felt like something too highly personal to share, plus I again kept thinking, what the fuck is wrong with you? Everyone else is living the dream and you aren't even able to do that. Their exuberance for life only served to make me feel even more isolated and different.

One Sunday morning before I went off to university, Mum and I had a brief discussion where the word depression was first used. In some ways using the term was a release, a relief even, but it was also scary and painful – saying it out loud made it real and once it had been said, there was no going back. The genie was out of the bottle. Looking back, I think it would have been better if we had delved deeper and spoken more about what was going on and what it actually meant to be depressed. I think the reason we didn't was that there was an element of embarrassment from us both and certainly shame on my part, no matter how misplaced. I kept thinking that even though the symptoms fit, surely I didn't actually have *that*, did I? I think we were in denial and also fearful, rightly so as it turned out, of what opening that particular can of worms might mean.

My enthusiasm for going to university was low. I kept waiting for the excitement to kick in. It didn't. It did, however, feel like I was doing what was expected of me, especially when literally one hundred per cent of my peer group were going. I was also short on other options and it felt easier to go along with the great plan rather than rail against it – even if I had had the energy to do so. I believed I could outrun the issue of my depression by going off to Southampton. Actually it was more blind hope than belief that my brain would kick into gear.

By the time the word depression was first used in our house the possibility was already buried deep in my consciousness, but saying it out loud was a whole other ball game. When Mum brought it up I just wanted her to shut up. It was too hard to talk about. I didn't *want* to talk about it or acknowledge it. It was more than I could cope with. I looked up the definition in an online dictionary shortly after that initial discussion and it said this:

Depression:

Noun

Feelings of severe despondency and dejection.

'Self-doubt creeps in and that swiftly turns to depression'

Melancholy, misery, sadness, unhappiness, sorrow, woe, gloom, gloominess, dejection, downheartedness, despondency, dispiritedness, low spirits, heavy-heartedness, moroseness, discouragement, despair, desolation, dolefulness, moodiness, pessimism, hopelessness

I read it a few times, then sat back in my chair, knowing that if I was ticking my responses it would have been:

Yes. Tick. To all of the above.

I chose to say nothing more, didn't really want to discuss it at length or in detail. I wasn't ready to make an admission of mental illness that was not only hard to hear, but also an idea that scared the shit out of me. If I pictured a depressed person, I imagined someone who was frail, weak and faded, all things that were and are very hard to imagine about yourself, as well as frightening.

Mental illness – it's like the very worst thing to have to admit about your brain and equally hard to admit to others. I also hoped, really hoped, it might be wrong. Maybe it wasn't depression, maybe it would go away, my mood would lift and I would start to live the dream and study Biology.

◆ ◆ ◆

Mum and Simeon drove me from Bristol and dropped me off among a sea of other cars and nervous-looking students. Some, I noticed, were already pairing up as mates and I felt the flickering of uncertainty; how did you get to be one of those people? The ones with the chat, who could do small talk and make plans for beers with complete strangers? It was alien to me. I did what I do best and kept my head down. The car was packed with new pillows, a duvet and various other shite from Ikea to try to make the bland, depressing rooms look less bland and depressing. I remember Mum faffing around in the small room, filling the space, organising books on to the windowsill, putting pens in the pen pot and laying a bright rug on the floor. Her presence and constant stream of reassuring chatter as she unwrapped stuff made the room seem even smaller. It annoyed me and was typical; I knew she'd be thinking that if she could make my room look 'nice', make it look like any other student room in any movie or sales pamphlet, then there was a chance I might behave like any other student. She just didn't get it. And this pissed me off more than I was prepared to say. She had always had this 'fix-it' tendency and I knew it came from a good place, but on that particular day it was, from my perspective, like trying to put a plaster on a gunshot wound and it bothered me that she couldn't see that, didn't get it. It showed me, as if proof were needed, that she didn't understand how depression isn't about the outside; it's about the inside.

I think I lost my temper and asked her to stop fussing and to go home. She had done enough, from stocking up the tiny kitchen cupboard to shoving all kinds of shit on to my noticeboard, and all I wanted was to be left alone. To sleep.

Mum cried – shock, horror – but they left, and I immediately sank down on to the mattress and closed my eyes. It was at that point that I began to realise that this feeling, the dark creep of exhaustion, did not care where the mattress on which I lay my head was or about the post code in which I lived, it didn't care for much apart from consuming me. I think in hindsight I knew in that second as I closed my eyes that my relationship with depression was not coming to an end as I might have hoped; in fact it felt like the perfect environment for it to thrive. But, again, I didn't say anything, partly because I did not want it to be true and partly because my parents had not yet reached the car park in the halls of residence. But mainly because this was my first hour on campus and I thought this gloomy scenario might be a bit premature and, it sounds stupid, because a small part of me still really, really hoped that I was wrong. But I was scared. Really scared. I wanted to run. I wanted to sleep. I wanted to be at home. I wanted company. I wanted to be alone. I didn't know what I wanted. I felt completely overwhelmed by the whole experience.

I stayed in my room for the whole of that day and night, pretty much just lying on the bed. My energy levels were low. I listened through the window to the chatter of student life and the shouts and hollers of those making plans, and I remember thinking that if I could press a button and disappear I would. And yet I did not equate this thought with suicide, not at that point. But maybe that was the start of it. I don't know. I felt a little remote from what was going on, a bit like a bystander, even though I was in the thick of it; there was noise and bustle all around and there was I, alone in my room.

After only a few days of living in the halls of residence, it became obvious that my unwillingness to go outside, social anxiety and exhaustion meant it was going to be very hard, if not impossible, to take care of my personal administration – things like laundry, cooking and cleaning. It felt easier to ignore it all and sleep. And so I did just that.

Ironically, I hauled my arse out of bed to attend introduction lectures about making the most of student life and about what to do if you felt lonely. Socials were organised with the sole aim of getting people to mix. I think someone from a Christian group might have even brought me a sandwich, but it's all a bit muddled in my mind. I just know I was lost, more lost if that's possible, and I honestly didn't know what to do.

I settled into life at uni as best I could. Most of my school friends saw leaving home as their chance to start living and experimenting. Freedom! For me it was the exact opposite; it was my chance to sink into the dark hole that I had been peering into for quite a while. And I could do so without the fear of Mum or Simeon climbing the stairs and poking their head around the door to check on me or bring me a cold drink. So I guess that in itself was a form of freedom, just a very different one from that of my peers. I didn't have to pretend or even try, and to be frank that was a relief.

My accommodation was a single room along a quiet, artificially lit corridor that looked like any nondescript office block on any out-of-town industrial estate. The images of uni life that had been burned into my subconscious via prospectuses and social media had promised so much: fun and camaraderie, parties and sex. Well, if this was a party, it was the kind organised by your nan where hardly anyone turns up and the only thing on offer is orange squash and everyone is collected by their parents at 7 p.m. prompt.

Life on my corridor was . . . well, there wasn't much life on my corridor. I had thought a single room with its own bathroom would be good for privacy and quiet, but it was actually quite lonely. I spent the first few days cloistered away on my floor listening to the quiet comings and goings of others, but I knew if I didn't head out of the room and force myself to mix then that loneliness was only going to intensify.

Mum, Simeon, Nan and Grandad kept calling or texting and asking excitedly, 'Have you made friends? Are you having a nice time?'

Their questions, no matter how well intentioned, felt like a pressure. It was easier to say 'yes' and let their sighs of relief echo down the line. At least they would be getting a good night's sleep based on the lie. But their relief only further confirmed that my isolation was another failure. I felt very much like the boy with his back to the class.

It took every ounce of confidence I have ever possessed to leave the room and venture to the floor below and knock on the door of a shared flat that sounded like they were having a party. But I did it. These people were strangers, but at some level I knew if I didn't get out of that room it would set a pattern that would be no good for me. I felt like I stood out, awkward. This was in no way down to the hosts, who were kind and welcoming; it was all down to my messed-up brain.

The people in this flat became people to get drunk with, go to nightclubs with and even play rugby with, although after one or two sessions I was in so much physical discomfort that yet again my body thwarted my desire to get involved with the sport I love. I might now have been at university but this fact didn't piss me off any less.

At this point I was not entirely lost to depression, there were some days that were brighter than others, when I felt able to inter-act and the world did not seem so bleak. I would go to lectures and be a 'normal' student. These periods of 'normality' could last anything from one day to a week or so. They gave me hope.

Looking back, I can see that I self-medicated with alcohol. I drank a lot. Not every day, but I would conservatively guess I was boozing for four days out of seven. I can't properly remember exactly what I drank or how much, but I know it was an obscene amount and was a mix of spirits and beer. And I can't lie: there were a handful of hilarious nights out when life felt good. When drunk, I felt able to socialise and mix with my peers like anyone else of a similar age and position. It's strange for me to think that anyone who met me on those nights out would have seen a confident, outgoing person and would have had no idea of what I was going through or how I lived. I liked being able to live in the moment without depression anchoring me. Most importantly, I felt able to cope. I also liked the oblivion of passing out after drinking too much, the escape a relief from the anxiety that dogged me every day.

I had long held the idea that to win a place at university and study the one subject I loved would be brilliant. The reality wasn't quite like that and the disappointment dragged me further down. I went to a couple of lectures at the beginning of the term and even made a stab at some coursework, but that was it. Looking back, I can see that the level of teaching at Southampton was first class but I wasn't in the right frame of mind to capitalise on it, preferring to sleep and hide away rather than engage. And unlike at school no one gave a shit whether you were present or not and I was grateful for it. I did the bare minimum and got through the term, again on residual knowledge from my past studies, thankful to Dr P and lucky that I had such an understanding of my topic. I knew, however, that this would not get me very far in the long run and I think I had mentally accepted that it would all blow up eventually – it was just a case of when, not if. This feeling of waiting to be exposed did nothing to help my mental state.

The end-of-year exams came around quickly. I fielded calls from my parents, reassuring them, as I had every week since they had dropped me off, that everything was peachy. It was a terrible time for me and I did my level best to hide it. I felt under the most enormous pressure and stayed awake for the best part of forty hours, revising, cramming, drinking coffee, taking small naps and studying some more. I would limp to the exam hall, take the exam feeling like death and almost crawl home to collapse and sleep. The sleep that came after these almost manic episodes of crazy work and study, trying to catch up, would last for hours and then, depending on when the next exam was, I would wake and start the whole horrible process again. I can vividly remember my hands shaking so vigorously during one exam I struggled to control the mouse, just another indication of how lack of sleep compounded with stress and high caffeine doses were taking their toll on my mental and physical health.

I didn't know what was happening. I felt out of it. I was confused, dazed and scared. I couldn't get into a routine. I continued to socialise at night time with my new friends and I don't think they were aware of the state I was in. It felt like the world had been tilted and I was clinging to a narrow ledge with my fingertips, but I knew it was only a matter of time before I had to let go and hurtle down and down. I thought about the previous summer and was rightly wary of the fall.

There was only one thing I dreaded more than spending day after day in my bland, messy room in Southampton and having to take exams, and that was having to go home and pretend.

But this too, I knew, was inevitable.

Chapter Eleven

AMANDA

'LIFE ON TRACK'

'Happiness was but the occasional episode in a general drama of pain.'

Thomas Hardy

The day we left Josh in Southampton was a tough one. Simeon drove me home in tears. It was about as far from the movie farewell with a cheery grin as I could imagine. The temptation to call and check on him was strong, but as Simeon pointed out it was all about giving him independence and the confidence to be alone and it would do him no favours if I was hounding him every few minutes as if I did not believe he could cope. He was right of course, not that it made it any easier or made me worry any less.

I remember saying to Simeon when we arrived home, 'You read some terrible things about kids at university, you don't think he'd do anything stupid, do you?'

And he looked at me across the table and said, 'Like what?'

And I couldn't say the words, '*Take his own life, kill himself.*' And so instead I stared at him until he placed his hand on my arm and said, 'No way. He would never do anything like that. He's a smart kid.'

At the end of that first day, Josh sent a text around bedtime to say, 'All good' – this was his customary reply and I slept a whole lot better to see those two little words flash up on my screen.

And it did get easier. A little. The more time passed without any emergency call or disaster threatening, the more I, as a mum, and we, as a couple, relaxed. Simeon and I started to take advantage of the gap in our headspace and grew closer, spending more time together, undertaking book tours, walking around the Bristol docks of an evening and not letting the kids be our only topic of conversation. The boys going away to study proved to be a sharp learning curve for me. Ben was at a local college, but never home. He enjoyed a wonderful social life and if he wasn't socialising he was playing team sports. On our regular trips to Southampton or if Josh came home for the weekend, he certainly didn't take to his bed. His calls were short, our regular chats perfunctory, but he said he was doing well, going out and meeting people. I believed him and in tandem with this, began to think that maybe the use of the word 'depression' had been a bit premature and I was thankful for it, relieved even. It was at this point that I let my guard down. He gave no real hint that he was in difficulty and I remember hoping that his eagerness to end our chats was because he had something pressing or fun calling him and that thought made me so happy.

This new life with my kids spreading their wings forced me to look at that fine line between providing a safety net for the boys, letting them know we were there as and when they needed us, and mollycoddling them. I can't say finding the balance was easy. I think I still believed, or wanted to believe, that they needed me, but that's much more about my attachment to my mothering role than about them. It was also a bitter thought that Josh seemed to be coping a lot better away from me. Was I part of the problem? I found that hard to consider.

I still greeted every contact or lack thereof with an element of concern, frequently asking: do you think the boys are okay? To which Simeon would nod. But as the weeks passed my worry calmed and it's fair to say I felt entirely optimistic as Josh approached the end of his first year at Southampton University. Not only optimistic, but buoyed up, happy even! Everyone had said, and I agreed, that if he could make it through the first year without incident then the rest would be plain sailing, and Josh was clearly thriving. My proof for this being that he had not run home to seek the refuge of his bed, he was instead staying at university and seemed to be embracing student life.

I was happy that things were finally working out for our boy and I agreed with Simeon that we had nothing to worry about. It was during this, Josh's first year of university, that we finally popped a cork and raised our glasses. With both my boys settled, I slept easy. I was so very proud of how Ben had established a life at college and of the kind young man he was becoming and of how Josh had overcome the most horrible time. I didn't confess, even to myself, the jolt of concern I felt when I saw posts about Josh on social media, never posted by him, but always named by a friend. In every single photograph I saw of Josh he was drunk, lopsided, leaning, bloated, bleary-eyed and with his arms around strangers in a similar state or on at least one occasion, actually unconscious.

Simeon and I discussed it and agreed that whilst we should look out for his drinking and chat to him when he was home next about things that were habit-forming, we were content, relieved that he had made a new friendship group. We justified the slightly unsettling posts with the reasoning that surely all students drank a lot, didn't they? Wasn't this the exact time for experimentation?

The time to get it out of his system. Isn't it what we had wished for when he had taken to his bed and refused to engage with anyone? My God, the thought of *that* boy, the one sleeping in the foetal position for hours on end, the very idea that he might be in a nightclub, having fun – well, that would have been the dream! Plus, in addition to our weekly chats, Josh spoke to Simeon with greater frequency and we travelled down to Southampton to take him for lunch or a coffee at least once a month. As his mum, I was confident that if anything had been amiss, I would have seen it. I would have *felt* it . . .

The one thing I had always prided myself on was my closeness to Josh, my good parenting skills and the fact that my instincts where he was concerned were usually right. These beliefs were, I felt, validated when the results of his first-year exams came in. Josh had scored highly and I was so pleased for him. Our boy was on his way to getting a degree. Life was on track – more than on track, life was brilliant!

When Josh arrived home for the long summer break before starting the second year in September, he seemed to be in fairly good spirits, a little quiet and a little tired, sure, but we knew he had been burning the candle at both ends and were glad that he was getting a little down time. He, Ben and a group of friends had decided months before to go travelling. We encouraged this, telling them to take advantage of the holidays before the demands of bills and rent plus a lack of time, made such things harder. I have been raised with the belief that the very best thing you can do in life is to go out and talk to people, all people. That's how we learn, break down barriers and become part of a wider community. It's something that if finances had allowed I would have loved to have done in my youth, but the most I could hope for was a day trip to Boulogne-sur-Mer on a hovercraft with a forty-minute window to wander along a windy beach before the coach took us back to the port.

I wanted it to be different for my boys and was excited for them as well as hopeful that it might give Josh the shot in the arm of confidence he needed, a chance to learn about himself and his place in the big wide world. With a route set, they were going to visit Cambodia, Thailand, Vietnam and Malaysia – taking in sights, partying a little and meeting up with other mates who were also travelling. I envied them both the experience and opportunity.

They were home for a couple of weeks before we watched them pack rucksacks with all the essentials and the night before they left we sat down for supper. The boys were chatty, excited, but we could tell that their outward confidence was underpinned with a measure of caution. Quite right too; going off on a life adventure like this was not without possible dangers, but we figured overcoming these dangers and the things that would inevitably go wrong was all part of their learning.

At the end of his semester we had loaded all of Josh's belongings into the car and moved him from his room in the halls of residence into a very grotty shared student house, which was empty and in a run-down area of town. Josh had been allocated a room in the roof, which seemed fine on paper, until we discovered that at well over six foot, he could not stand up in it. We dumped his belongings into a small room on a lower floor and with plenty of rooms for all the occupants, naively figured that people would simply grab a room and a much shorter person would take the loft room. They would all then live life in harmony.

How wrong we were! That very night before they left to go travelling and as we were sitting down to eat, I received a call from a very disgruntled student – apparently Josh had gone into the room allocated to this boy. Goodness me, that conversation was a shocker, emotions were running very high, and the only person who would suffer in the long term was Josh, who needed nothing less than this feeling of angst over his next year's accommodation. I watched his face sink and he announced that he didn't want to go travelling. He was adamant. That telephone call and subsequent fiasco over a bloody bedroom had made his anxiety rear its ugly, powerful head in ways we could not imagine.

I was furious and distressed in equal measure. This trip had been long planned and hard saved for and was his one chance to go and see a bit of the world. And yet there we were the night before he was due to board a plane with his currency in his wallet, passport and tickets in his pocket and clothes washed, ironed and rolled inside his backpack, trying to convince him that it would all be fine and that he shouldn't let some over-dramatic shouting deprive him of this once-in-a-lifetime trip. Simeon and I believed that if he didn't go, he would not only regret it, but it would reinforce the idea that this kind of adventure and fun was for other people and not him, not Josh, the boy who had sat with his back to the class. We urged him to go.

Was it the right decision? I don't know. I've thought about it a lot since. As his mum, I can only see all the small misjudgements that led up to him wanting to take his life. Stepping stones if you like, each one constructed from an incident, a word, an experience that led to that one awful November day in 2016.

When he agreed to go I felt immediately conflicted: how would he cope if they ran into difficulty? And what was the plan if we needed to get to him? I was loath to put the responsibility on Ben's shoulders, although, as it turned out, they ended up travelling separately for much of the time, heading to different countries. I think Ben found Josh hard to be with when he was low. Contact while they were away was understandably limited, but the messages that came back to us via text or the odd email were positive: 'ALL GOOD. HOSTEL FINE. SEE YOU SOON.'

Nothing to cause any real worry and yet nothing to suggest that this was turning out to be the best experience ever. But I think this slightly muted communication was what we had come to expect from Josh over the last year or so.

It was when he and Ben came back together from travelling after a couple of months away that I think the situation reached a new low. I had hoped, beyond hoped, prayed that he might come back with a spring in his step and a broad smile: energy for the year ahead, if you like, and a newfound enthusiasm for life. I figured, again naively (how many times do I have to write that word until the ping of shame ceases to fire around my gut?) that being away from home and university, travelling around was a chance for Josh to breathe . . . Again I can see that I was basing his travelling experience on my own mindset, knowing that when things feel like they are getting on top of me or I have a problem that needs to be untangled, a change of scenery or a walk on a beach does much to restore my equilibrium. It didn't seem to be the case with Josh.

I couldn't wait to get the boys home from their trip and to hear of all their adventures in countries I had never visited, and was genuinely looking forward to combing through countless pictures of temples, beaches, bars and the faces of strangers – enabling me to live the travels vicariously through them. I cooked a supper, put beer in the fridge and waited with a whoop of excitement in my gut for the boys to walk through the door . . .

Josh returned from his trip with an expression that was fraught and my heart sank. He gave a tight smile and said he had had a nice time. It all felt rather damp and lukewarm – and for the first time I began to understand that there was no place or experience that could make him happy. Ben, on the other hand, was glad to be home and had a new quiet confidence about him. He had, he assured us, had the *best* time, met some great people, seen some amazing things. And we all agreed it was no mean feat to have

120

travelled, overcome obstacles and made it safely home – heck, these were the same boys who in recent times had thought it okay to cook a pizza in a sideways toaster and saw nothing wrong in building rockets that they fired over the house, narrowly missing a neighbour's car. This in the time when they were closer, before Josh's illness set them on very different paths. Needless to say I was more than happy to have them home in one piece, seemingly with all disasters averted. I remember Josh's face very clearly, tanned and with his hair in need of a cut, unshaven and a little weary looking: from travelling I hoped. His eyes, I noted, were a little vacant.

But it soon transpired Josh was not just tired from travelling, once again he was beyond tired: exhausted. Both boys walked into the hallway and I kissed Ben and reached up to hold Josh in a hug, no mean feat, as Josh is six foot two. He placed his head on my shoulder and cried. I felt the stirrings of fear and was a little overwhelmed by his sadness, it made my tears spring too. The four of us stood awkwardly in the cramped space, all thoughts of celebration sucked from the atmosphere, and neither Simeon nor myself were quite sure of what to do next. In fact, this has been the one constant throughout Josh's struggle, the feeling of ineptitude and our matching expressions of utter bewilderment as our cogs turn and we hope and pray that when they stop we might be presented with a solution in a light-bulb moment: a brilliant idea on how to tackle things. We are nearly five years on and, yes, we have done some things right, but we have also done some things wrong. And the cogs are still turning.

'It's okay, Josh . . .' I whispered, and these words now sounded like a lie in my ears too. He nodded, but I think we both knew that things were far, far from okay. One thing was for certain, there was no space in that weighted atmosphere for cold beer or a celebratory meal.

Both boys littered the house with their laundry, gifts, camping gear and all the lovely souvenirs they had collected – Josh gave me a tiny gold Buddha he had picked up from a street vendor near a temple. I still treasure it. Ben jumped into the shower and Josh slunk off to bed. I checked in on him an hour or so later – he was in a deep, deep sleep, his tanned skin looked grimy against the white sheets, not that it mattered, nothing did, only allowing my boy the rest he craved. I held the little fat Buddha in my palm and prayed. I prayed that he might wake feeling better, calmer and with more light behind his eyes. Buddha did not grant my wish, nor any of the other gods I also mentioned in my prayers, figuring it best to cover all bases.

And this time, I did feel it, could sense that things were not great. The trouble was, I didn't know what to do about it, didn't want to upset his plans to return to Southampton and start his second year, didn't want to take the shine from his end-of-year exam results which were still fresh in our minds, and I didn't want to think for a moment that he might sink back into the self-imposed exile that had been so hard to witness during his last year of school. I truly believed that the previous summer's melancholy had been a blip and clung to the facts as I believed them to be: that Josh had had a wonderful first year at Southampton with a roaring social life and great exam results and was having fun as he found his feet. I wanted to believe this. I so, so wanted it to be true.

He once again took to his bed.

And I was heartbroken.

It felt like his degree course was in jeopardy, along with the plan for the next couple of years – a plan that had given us all a welcome sense of security. If he didn't go back to university, what then? I still believed that the routine of studying and spending time with his peers while slowly growing in independence was the best thing for him.

Chapter Twelve

JOSH

'A TICKET TO TRAVEL'

'The loneliest moment in someone's life is when they are watching their whole world fall apart, and all they can do is stare blankly.'

F. Scott Fitzgerald

Travelling was another fine example of living what everyone told me was the dream: my best life. What an opportunity! Your time is your own, you lucky bastard. You'll meet new people and see the world, sit on a beach, drink a cold one and bob about on warm seas with like-minded individuals from across the globe, all lucky enough to have that ticket to travel.

And I tried, I did, but it was a lie. It wasn't the dream, not for me. It was anything but. I felt nothing but anxiety at the prospect of going to another country and then another country, checking into faceless airports and trying to figure out flickering departure boards while sitting in air-conditioned chaos. It was hard at this point to remember the time when I had looked forward to this trip – now it felt more like I was there through a fear of missing out. It all felt like an upheaval, a hassle, or worse, crowding on to stifling hot buses where there was no room for personal space or boundaries, where the world was literally in my face. Making friends with strangers over and over while we sat around zinc-topped tables, trying with varying degrees of success to decipher wipe-clean menus. And we all wore matching tans and cotton shorts, as we nimbly slid the labels from ice-cold bottles of beer, waiting for our turn to regale the exact same story everyone else had to tell: 'Vietnam was beautiful, Thailand hot, Malaysia expensive . . . Goa sounds like fun.'

I tried and failed not to sound like a wanker, but I did not have the energy to put a spin on events that might set me apart nor any desire to use my smarts or funnies. And now, years later, each night I spent travelling, preserved in memory, merges with every other. The groups that gathered in the hostels shared tales that were boring to me: bland stories told in unfamiliar bars in a variety of countries, but all looking out over the same shadowy shorelines. Laughter rippled like a Mexican wave among whichever group I was with, but I could only nod and drink, thinking not about the anecdote or what to say next, but fixated on packing and unpacking, anxious about the imaginary loss of documents, concerned over timescales, currency and language barriers, even when people were being friendly. I just wished they would leave me alone. I wished everyone would leave me alone. Ben and I split up. He went off to Vietnam while I headed to Cambodia to see Angkor Wat, and it was worth the trip, even in my fogged state I knew it was a very special place.

At some level I felt guilty. I knew that I should be enjoying the experiences more, and that there were a million people my age who would bite my arm off for the same opportunity, many of them back home saving every penny in the hope of one day getting a ticket that booked them a seat at this table. Yes, millions of people . . . I just wasn't one of them. It wasn't rare for me to look at those I travelled with and feel so lonely I wanted to run, had my crappy joints allowed. I felt like an imposter in this incredible life, an imposter who was determined to sabotage even the most amazing of experiences. It meant I could barely relate to those I travelled with and did not feel the same levels of elation or wonder at the incredible sights I captured with my camera, when I could be bothered. I was no more than an extension of the lens, but I did not have awareness to look beyond what I was framing.

Again a feeling of hollowness swamped me. If anything, the trip felt like a chore, like work. I can't believe I have written that, but it's the truth. How ridiculous – there I was in paradise and all I could think of was climbing into bed and shutting the whole world out. Of course it wasn't the trip that was at fault. It wasn't the people I travelled with and it certainly wasn't the incredible countries that welcomed me. The problem was me. Of course the problem was me! I did those places a great disservice, unintentionally, but the result was the same.

With the fog of depression and introspection now lifted a little, I often think about returning one day, without a camera and travelling alone to look and see and learn and appreciate the places I shuffled through, eyes fixed on the floor, numbed. I might even join a group around a table and share a cold beer. I might even have a tale or two to tell . . .

I arrived home in an exhausted daze. I remember Mum and Simeon were full of questions and I couldn't take it. I couldn't take what felt like an interrogation no matter how well meant and I didn't want to stand there and lie about my incredible life-changing adventure that had been anything but.

I think I got upset, really upset.

I know I went straight to bed.

And stayed there for the rest of the time I had at home, about three weeks.

Hiding away.

I remember my grandparents visiting and wanting to know all about my trip and I knew they were waiting to hear great stories about the places I had seen, but everything, even talking to them, felt like a chore. This just made me feel guilty because I understood that their joy was in knowing I was happy, having a great time, but I was not happy or having a great time and I couldn't pretend. I could see that my lack of enthusiasm and energy disappointed them but I couldn't change it. I didn't know how. I had even forgotten how to pretend.

It felt like no time at all until we were once again packing up the car to return to Southampton for my second year at university. I was pretty numb. Mum and Simeon spent the best part of my time at home tiptoeing around me as if I was made of glass. And actually they were right. I was made of glass: so fragile that one knock and I might have shattered. Their whispers in the hallway, slow knocks on the door and soft tread into the room while I slept drove me crazy. Irritated me. More than once I heard Mum whisper, *I don't know what to do . . .* and I'd sink beneath the duvet thinking *join the club, Mandy*. I know I was impatient and sharp with them, withdrawn, and that obviously encouraged them to approach with greater caution and a nervous air, which only made me feel worse – it was a shit situation where the level of anxiety was sky high and we were locked in this kind of Chinese finger trap behaviour. A fucking nightmare.

They had decided after the whole accommodation fiasco that the shared house was not a good place for me to stay and certainly not the best environment to help my mental health, and so while I was away travelling they secured me a studio in a part of the city popular with students. The studio was nice on the inside: brand new and with its own kitchen and bathroom. They had kitted it out with a sofa and bookshelves, a decent bed, lamps, pictures and everything I might need in the kitchen, including glasses and plates and a coffee machine. I remember thinking that it was the kind of flat where someone might be able to cook and have mates over, if that person wasn't me who was determined not to invite anyone into my living space. It didn't feel like mine.

I went through the motions with Mum helping me unpack. I watched her position plants on the surfaces with instructions on how to care for them. I didn't listen. Her presence irritated the fuck out of me and it was a sharp reminder of how little things had changed for me since that first day of arriving in halls when she did the exact same thing. I guess this time I understood why a little more. She was trying to keep control of the things she could whilst the things she couldn't, my mental state, for example, stayed just out of reach. I just wanted her to leave me alone . . . so I could sleep. Ah yes, my old friend sleep, my security blanket, my happy (ish) place, my haven . . . sleep. It was all I could think about.

I remember her lingering nervously in the car park, standing on the gravel with her bag in her hands, preparing to drive home.

'Will you be okay, Joshy?'

'Yes.'

'Are you still a bit depressed, do you think?'

'I don't think so. No.'

'If you ever . . . if ever you want to talk to someone—'

'I don't.' I cut her short.

'But if you did.'

'I don't!' I really, really wanted her to go.

'What can I do to help you, Joshy?'

You can fuck off and leave me alone. My thoughts, but instead I said, 'Nothing.'

'Do you ever feel suicidal, Josh?' Her eyes searched mine like she was looking for clues.

It was a huge question, the biggest, and one I suppose I had expected her to ask sooner, not that I had planned how I might respond. When it came to it, it felt like the easiest thing to almost brush it off. But the truth was I *had* thought about it, not a lot, but it was, I knew, an option for me. And no more than that. I also knew that to admit as much would send Mandy into the stratosphere – and *that* I could not have coped with. It was easier to say what I did and watch her leave rather than have to deal with her inevitable hysteria.

'Don't be so stupid,' I might have shouted, and her smile was one of relief.

Tick.

Tick.

Tick.

Tick . . . Keep ticking the boxes, Joshy boy, and you can keep it all at bay. At least that was what I thought.

I didn't think my mum was stupid, far from it, but it was all about getting her to leave in a state that meant she wasn't going to fret or, worse, call me when she got home to have the conversation all over again . . . I couldn't handle the thought of that. In hindsight, her questioning and observations were forcing me to look at my mental state and that was the last thing I wanted to do, preferring, at that point, to bury my head in the sand. I was still trying to figure everything out and at the same time keep those dark thoughts at bay.

Chapter Thirteen

AMANDA

'SIXTH SENSE'

'One word frees us from all the weight and pain of life.
That word is love.'

Sophocles

It was just before Josh returned to his new studio in Southampton for the start of his second year that Simeon and I discussed at length how to proceed, understanding that he was now an adult and in control of his own destiny and not wanting him to feel disenfranchised, but on the other hand he was still our son and we needed to know how best to help him. We figured the only way to do that was by trying to gain a clearer picture of where Josh was at and what he might be going through. Having seen his lack of energy and the state in which he had returned from travelling it was time to face some truths: Josh might not actually be coping as well at uni as he made out. I was wary of him being packed back off to Southampton without our support network and made the uncomfortable decision to contact Josh's professor in Southampton. This action was not something I undertook lightly. It felt sneaky, underhand, and I knew Josh would have been furious had he known. With his confidence at an all-time low and anxiety snapping at his heels, I recognised the importance of Josh feeling in control and also that any action taken without his consent, especially undertaken to glean information *about* him, was the very opposite of putting him in control.

It felt uncomfortable, but that was just too bad. I wanted to know if the university had any concerns about Josh or if any alarm bells were ringing. I wanted to know if there had been any depressive episodes, and in all honesty I wanted to talk to someone who could have seen this behaviour before in young students and might, just might, be able to give me some advice that could help us all. I figured that with insight and confirmation I could maybe put wheels in motion to help Josh get through whatever lay ahead. I carefully composed an email, explaining that I understood that the communication was possibly overstepping a boundary and that she was probably duty-bound not to disclose any personal information, but was there anything, *anything* at all she could tell me that might help us gain a clearer picture of what was going on with Josh? The wording was painstakingly thought out as I tried desperately to hide the growing feeling of hysteria in my gut. What I actually wanted to do was drive to Southampton and grab his teacher by the lapels and scream, 'Help me! Help us. What's going on with my son? What can I do? Tell me what to do!' But of course I didn't.

The prompt reply was short, polite and professional, letting me know that she was not able to discuss or disclose any information about a student without the student's prior agreement.

That was it. No room for manoeuvre or further discussion.

I let my finger hover over the keyboard . . .

Thank you for your reply, I began. *Okay, I understand, I do, but . . . but . . . what if it's a case of life or death? What if it might help my boy's mental health? What if it means he might stick at his degree and not drop out?* (And yes, I did use the term 'dropping out' back then before I had given it as much thought as I have today.)

I crafted the reply, still being polite, still trying to appeal to the woman's better nature whilst understanding that her hands were tied with administrative rope that was strong no matter how sharp the emotional knife I wielded. I pressed send while glancing at the little Buddha . . . but the second response was just as business-like and disappointing. It was quite clear that no matter what the circumstance, without Josh's explicit permission the university could not and would not talk to me.

I have thought about this long and hard, slicing and dicing the state of affairs as it was at the time in nearly every UK university and trying to make sense of it. It's a tough one, far from cut and dried, and I appreciate the complexity of where an emotional and sometimes desperate request has to be tempered with the greater, more logical approach of a system that is there to protect the majority. Data protection is a thorny and ever-expanding issue in these digital times where the safety and privacy of an individual online has never been more important. I know it's vital for students to be assured that their private information is just that. Plus, we are talking about students who are no longer kids, but adults with all the privileges and rights that come from being over eighteen. Who has the right to access their data without their permission? I get it. I am also aware that not all parents or guardians would use information garnered in this way for the good. Indeed, we know that it is unauthorised access to personal data, usually by those with dark intent, that reveals the sinister and sometimes dangerous results of not containing and protecting data.

My problem – actually frustration would be a better word – is that notwithstanding how important it is for these young adults to break out from the sheltered life of school and home to tread the path to adulthood, the leap from schoolboy to adult student is a marked one, huge in fact! And not only for the students – it's a fairly hefty emotional and physical hurdle for their parents too. I am delighted that change is afoot and many universities have been involved in developing The University Mental Health Charter, 'a Charter for university mental health in partnership with a range of leading charities and Higher Education bodies . . . rewarding those institutions that demonstrate good practice, make student and staff mental health a university-wide priority and deliver improved mental health and well-being outcomes.'[9] The Charter also undertakes to explore the key issue of whether an opt-in requirement for universities could be considered, so they could have permission to share information on student mental health with parents or a trusted person.

In many of the tragic cases of student suicide, the issue of contact with the parents and information-sharing is cited as something that needs to be looked at. The BBC News reported on Ben Murray, a student at Bristol University, who died in May 2018. At his inquest his father said, 'If a fresher who has worked hard to get A levels doesn't turn up you should get in touch. And they should have notified us, the family.' Mr Murray said the couple 'had no idea' anything was wrong and were 'distressed' the university did not do more after they identified him as 'a no-show'.[10] He added that Ben had previously told staff he was feeling 'anxious' and 'was unwell', but they 'failed to remember this when dismissing him', and similarly in the *Guardian*, on 22 January 2019, Natasha Abrahart's father spoke movingly about the effect of his daughter's suicide. Natasha was a twenty-year-old second-year physics student and a keen musician who enjoyed indoor climbing and baking cakes. He found email correspondence between his daughter and the university in which she disclosed suicidal thoughts. 'Up until that point we had been thinking that this tragedy had come about because she had not confided in anyone. But she had tried to get help,' he says.[11]

I wholeheartedly endorse a system where students can 'opt in' to allow the university to contact a parent or guardian if there are legitimate concerns over a student's mental health. What a wonderful thing!

There was no such scheme in place for Josh and without the opportunity to 'opt in' and having drawn a blank in trying to make contact with the university, I had to trust in the system and hope that if and when our son needed us, he would shout. I missed Ben, of course I did, but with Josh it was different. I didn't only miss him, I feared for him too. But how much to intervene and voice those concerns? It came back to that old balancing act – trying to strike the right level of support and encouragement while at the same time providing some kind of safety net. I thought we would be good at this, parenting from a distance. I thought I had a handle on things. But the lack of access to information was a huge obstacle for us to overcome when trying to support a child with mental health issues.

The fact is when Josh left school and before The University Mental Health Charter, a pupil effectively finished school in June or July, leaving the only system and culture they had ever known. A system where if they missed a lesson, failed to hand in a project, got injured on the sports field or there were wider pastoral care issues, you could be sure of a phone call, a letter home or at the very least that one of the teaching staff would be on hand to deal with the situation. This meant that if we were lucky, the care of our children in the school system was a dual thing, recognising that it takes an *academic village* to help raise a child . . . But for Josh and many others like him, a mere eight or twelve weeks after leaving school that same child could falter, become isolated, depressed even, self-harm, fail to attend a lecture or could get into any number of difficulties and you the parent had absolutely no line of sight of the issue and therefore no way of helping/supporting the person you love in their time of need.

It was my experience that on one day I was largely responsible for my son's well-being, playing an active role and responding to shared information and then suddenly on the next I was cut off. Completely cut off. And for a man like Josh that proved near fatal. I am not suggesting that parents be party to the same level of information as when their children are at school, i.e. a school report – nothing like! And I suspect that in most cases there would be no need at all for communication between already overstretched university staff and a student's respective parent/guardian. But I am glad things are changing, heartened at the thought that with the express understanding that *if* the need should arise, any concerns as to the welfare of a student can be shared and dealt with in a much more holistic way.

I believe the silo mentality and organisation of some universities needs to change. Often there is little cross-faculty communication and certainly no sharing of information with other services or indeed the families of those who might be in crisis. It is, to my mind, the exact opposite of a system that has a moral, if not legal responsibility to provide the best safety net for students in their care. We hear too often that for some, sadly, the cohesive approach and an agreement to share information comes too late and is offered retrospectively. In several of the cases where students have taken their own lives, warning signs, even direct admissions from the students themselves that they were in danger or struggling, were not shared or passed on. For some families it was only at the inquest into the tragic death of their loved ones that they found out that the person they had lost did indeed reach out or ask for help . . . I can only imagine how hard that must be to deal with. And again, the irony is that for the want of a few months and a different system, i.e. school life – that help would have been on hand and all concerns passed on.

I have chatted to many friends with children of a similar age, discussing the reality of empty nest syndrome. Not for one moment did I think I would feel it. I was busy leading a full life and had made so many plans that could come to fruition once I was no longer beholden to the school run, like waking without an alarm, taking up yoga, getting a dog . . . So it was quite a shock how much I missed the school run and the vague feeling of redundancy that I felt without it. I was more than a little relieved to know I was not the only parent who had wandered along the dimly lit hallway in the dark of night and into the empty bedrooms of my kids, to lay my head on their pillow and inhale the scent of them before having a good old cry. Odd really, as I was certain it would be the scent of my boys in all their fragrant forms that I really would not miss. All joking aside, I missed their noise. I missed their presence. I missed that overwhelmingly reassuring feeling of knowing the people I loved were safe and sound each night under one roof.

The teacher I communicated with, seeking information, was not a bad person, quite the opposite, she even signed off all communications kindly, and – without making too many assumptions – it felt like she wished she could tell me more. And in truth, I wished she could have.

I was not confident in raising the topic with Josh, knowing that in his current closed state he would simply ask to be left alone and repeat that he was 'fine!' when it was clear to all who came into contact with him that he was anything but. I eventually asked if he might like me to speak to one of his faculty staff, without telling him I had already tried, and knowing the only way to have the dialogue with the institution was with his permission. He shook his head vehemently and knitted his brows, 'No! No way!' came his emphatic, angry reply.

The manner of his response only added to my worry that all was not well and I began to wonder what exactly Josh was hiding. Again my thoughts returned to the big dark secret that might lurk in his cupboard, and I tried to reassure him in any number of ways that there was nothing he could do or say that would ever, ever change the way we felt about him and that he was free to talk to us about anything, anything! He stared at me blankly, eyes wide like a rabbit in the headlights. I decided not to push it, figuring that at that moment Josh just needed to know he could rely on me no matter what.

I felt sick about leaving Josh alone in that studio we had rented for him in Southampton. We had hauled his stuff over there while he was travelling, knowing how quickly places got snapped up and having decided there was no way he could stay in the grotty student house in a room he could not stand up in. This, however, was a nice space and one I knew I would have loved at a similar age, a fabulous den with all mod cons.

Josh, however, seemed a little less than impressed with the flat and everything we had filled it with to ensure a smooth glide path into life alone for the first time outside of his uni residence and away from home. I couldn't quite put my finger on why. Sixth sense? Maybe. A sense of foreboding? Possibly. All I could do was hope. I had to truly hope and pray that he was going to flourish because I could not see another route, another outcome. He wouldn't open up to me, would not open up to a professional no matter how many times we suggested this very thing. We made recommendations, reminded him of the importance of eating right, getting out into daylight, walking, going to the gym, swimming and seeing his friends, all the things we hoped would lift his mood. It was like living in a desperate limbo where the foundation was shaky and we had no idea what we were dealing with. I had to trust Josh to be truthful when discussing his emotions and how he was feeling, because I had nothing else.

Ironically, my career was going from strength to strength and at first I would sit on TV panels or sofas smiling my way through interviews and talking about the plots of my stories, but always with Josh at the back of my mind. In a short space of time I was then bringing out a couple of books a year and they were flying straight to the top of the charts – it was and is the most wonderful feeling and one I still feel so very thankful for. I thought about my early years at school: announcing that I wanted to write books and the look of derision cast in my direction by my teacher – the one who was sharp and spiky – and her particular expression that knocked the confidence from my internal thoughts and the ambition from my dreams: *You? Write a book? Ha!*

Turns out she was right. I could not write *a* book. I could not stop at one, but I might stop at one hundred, who knows? My TV appearances became more regular and I discovered my spiritual home of radio. I was busier than ever and I think being so wrapped up in my writing with a hefty schedule for both the editing and delivery of novels and the PR schedule that went with each book, both in the UK and all over the world, it's fair to say that I took my eye off the ball. I think I wanted to believe that Josh was fine so I could concentrate on the job in hand – that of writing the very best books and making them the most successful they could be. There were nights, I am sure, when I fell asleep thinking about my latest book or planning the next one, and it feels horrible to consider that I might have mentally relegated what Josh was going through whilst applying myself to furthering my career. But I fear it's the truth. I figured that if I could make a success of my work then financial security would follow and I could concentrate on making life good for Josh, for Ben, for all of us.

Chapter Fourteen

Josh

'The very worst day'

'Teach me to live, that I may dread the grave as little as my bed.'

Thomas Ken

I was midway through my second year at university and still living alone in the studio flat.

My mental health declined to such an extent that I chose to withdraw from my social life. From everything. There was no sudden catalyst for this, no notable event. It just all suddenly felt like too much. I no longer wanted to be in the company of my drinking buddies, didn't want to see anyone or even drink.

I shut myself off from student life in every way possible. I was on autopilot. And like a robot I went through the motions, doing the bare minimum in every aspect of my life and shutting out the outside world. I watched the odd lecture online, read the occasional article, sent a couple of emails promising that course work would be forthcoming. I ate and drank, made the odd phone call to keep the worried messages from Mum and Simeon at bay. As I say, the bare minimum. So to the outside world I was functioning, just, but the reality was on the inside I had started to lose my grip. It was scary.

In the last year I had become an expert liar, masking how low I felt. I acted for my family when they made contact – I found it hard to open up and be truthful for fear of making them worry and being a burden on their busy lives. The shame factor and stigma of mental illness was for me greater than my ability to ask for the help I desperately needed. I knew I was slipping further into the abyss but was at a loss as to how to stop it.

'How are you feeling, Joshy?'

'Fine.' *Tick.*

'Do you need anything?'

'No.' *Tick.*

'Are you going to lectures?'

'Yes.' *Tick.*

'Have you seen your friends?'

'Yes.' *Tick.*

'Do you want us to come down and see you? Do you want to come home?'

'No.'

In fact, the last one was not a lie.

I did not want to see anyone, particularly those close to me who had no clue of what I was going through, and I honestly thought I would never go home again. This didn't concern me.

My parents would call and ask benign questions and offer pointless solutions that I knew were the worst kind of sticking plaster. The kind of thing that might have made them feel better in that they had a need to do 'something' but actually everything they suggested only proved my theory that they had no concept of what I was going through and that in turn made me feel even more alone.

I have struggled with how best to describe it, but if my brain switched off during my A levels then during this time and over a matter of months something new happened. It was like the colour had been switched off in the world. It was a gradual thing and so there was never a point where I opened my eyes and was shocked. It was more like slowly turning down the colour on a TV until one day the picture is entirely muted in tones of silver, grey and black. I do remember walking along the street one day and thinking that the world looked gloomy, dull, but it kind of suited me and I never thought to ask anyone if that was the colour they saw too or if it was just me.

Attending lectures never entered my head: that was for another life, another time and other people. I declined every invitation to meet up with friends, until they inevitably dwindled and they stopped asking or checking in on me and eventually the phone practically stopped ringing. This was not something I reflected on; I was glad not to have the distraction, the pressure, and felt free in a way. The best defence against having to interact with others was to keep my phone switched off or on silent and hide it from view. It worked. I liked the peace, the quiet. I was as isolated as I could be, bar a weekly conversation with Mum and Simeon where I went through the motions:

'How are you doing, Joshy?'

'Fine.' *Tick.*

'Do you want to come home?'

'No.' *Tick.*

'I'm going to Australia for work, will you be okay?'

'Yep.' *Tick.*

Getting out of bed was hard but one day I made an appointment to see one of my professors and sloped into the building where students gathered in huddles, laughing, wearing backpacks

140

heavy with books and drinking coffee. I was wearing sweatpants and a grubby football shirt, my hair unwashed. The whole environment felt alien to me. I told him in the least amount of words, trying to get the whole ordeal over in the shortest amount of time so I could return to bed, that I was thinking of dropping out of my course, leaving university. It wasn't a snap decision exactly, but equally it wasn't something I had overly considered, weighing up all the pros and cons as you might expect for a decision of this magnitude. Nor did I talk it through with anyone or seek advice. Not only did my sense of isolation support the idea that it was my decision to make alone, but also it felt inevitable: of course I was going to leave, who had I been trying to kid? And once I saw it as this, it felt better just to get it done. One less thing to clutter up my brain. He replied with the fact that no one had seen me for months! His implication was clear: *and this would be different how?* I told him I was not doing so well but did not go into specifics. He made a note, nodded and showed me the door. I felt he was a little irritated by my lack of attendance, couldn't care less, and it only added to my feeling of low self-worth. Of course he didn't give a shit, why would he? It was only Josh.

There was no follow up. No suggestion of where I should go from here, no advice on who I should speak to or where I might get help should I need it. He was busy. I get it. Busy with students who wanted to be there. His phone was ringing, there was a queue of people outside his door and he was harried. I can now see that not only was I viewing the situation through the lens of depression, but I know that he was also a good bloke, simply too busy to give my decision any more thought. He was not a bad person, far from it, but was a symptom of a system where even the most dedicated are overstretched with administration and are chasing numbers and success like any other business. And I believe the mental health of staff and students alike is suffering because of it.

I left his room quietly and sank further still. I knew my actions were building to a conclusion, a pinnacle, I just didn't know what or how. It was about a week or so later that I told the university I was certain about leaving my course, dropping out, *finito*. Making the decision to quit was the first time in a while that I felt in control, and through the numbness I felt a small amount of relief at the thought of not having to return to lectures – or at least pretend to return to lectures – not having to get out of bed, not having to participate. In every sense I was done. No one in the faculty, or indeed the university, said anything to try to talk me out of it or ask why. No one made contact. Not that I would, in fairness, have been open about my reasons if they had. I avoided the weekly calls from Mum and Simeon and kept them at bay by firing off the odd one- or two-word text, 'All good.' It seemed to be enough.

I used to lie in bed in that little studio and I could hear the people in other flats talking, singing or arguing. The sound travelled through pipes and weirdly came out of the extractor fan above the hob. It was freaky and unnerving. Like I needed that on top of everything else. The Polish voices became invasive, a language I couldn't understand – were they talking about me? This paranoia was a new thing, but no less scary for that. And I remember checking with the odd visitor passing through that they could hear them too. I was relieved that they could.

The darkness was winning – that's the only way I can think to describe it – my field of vision getting narrower and narrower. Every aspect of my life felt like an enormous pressure. The stress of having got behind in my academic work, the stress of having decided to leave but not yet having told my family, the stress of trying to convince others that I was okay via that weekly text, even having to get out of bed and wash and dress, launder clothes, clean my teeth, speak to someone – all of these things took more energy than I had. Real life was suspended; it took every ounce of my effort to stay present. To not give up. Because I wanted to give up, I wanted to give in. I wanted the peace that eluded me. I was done.

There was a new and persistent thought that I had up until that point managed to keep at bay and it was this: I figured that suicide might be the answer. I kept it to myself, wrangling with the idea. And strangely the thought of death didn't frighten me. In fact, I welcomed it. All I wanted was to drift off to sleep without the nagging thought of having to wake. Eternal sleep. It was not only attractive but also felt necessary for me to find any kind of peace. I didn't really think of it in terms of life and death. I thought of it no more than in terms of a way to stop the overwhelming fatigue. It felt like an easy decision.

In the depths of my illness when I am lost to it, 3 a.m. is my favourite time. It comes with blissful quiet, knowing that the world doesn't expect anything of you, no one is going to call, no one is going to ask you to do something. It's just you and the universe in perfect stillness. I had created a room where it was 3 a.m. always, not thinking of the long-term effects this might have. It was almost as if my flat existed in a different space, like a boulder in a stream, stuck in stillness whilst time flowed around it. I can't clearly remember how many days and nights I spent in that studio room before I gave up mentally and gave up on life. Time meant nothing and I lost track of it, unaware if I'd been there for weeks or months. Sleep was so all-consuming that when I roused I didn't know if I'd slept for an hour or a day. I didn't know or care if it was day or night.

I remember Mum asking before she headed off to Australia to work on a TV show if a trip abroad might make me feel better? Did I want to get some sunshine? Her naivety was as frustrating as it was outstanding. I wanted to rage at her: did she still *really* think that my happiness lay in a place and all I had to do was travel there, sit on a beach or climb up a mountain and, hey presto, I would feel jolly or cured?

Jesus Christ, we had tried that and my travels had not seen me return a new man, full of the joys . . .

On the occasions that I spoke to Mum, Simeon, my grandparents or friends, I was convinced I heard small tuts under people's breath and could sense the slight shake of a head behind their smiles, and I got it. I knew what they were thinking: *What the fuck is going on with you? Lazy bastard. Why don't you get out of bed? Why don't you DO something?* And I could only avert my eyes and agree, yep, what the fuck is going on with me? I wish I knew.

It would have been pointless to try to explain the hell in which I lived and, besides, nothing mattered – not what anyone else said or thought, not even my life.

You would not think it possible to spend so many hours lying on a bed doing nothing, concentrating on every breath, every change in the light, every heartbeat, but that's what I did. Hours and hours and hours and hours just lying still and waiting . . . for what? I don't know – a thought, an escape, a feeling . . . Even my good friends from home and new friends from university got bored. I don't blame them. And, besides, I understood because *I* was bored with it. Bored and defeated. Everything felt pointless and every small particle of joy that had shone in my future, always just out of reach, was now dulled until even my future was grey and dark . . . The thought of having to rouse myself and face whatever lay ahead was more than I could stand. I wasn't up to it.

It is a hard thing to admit and even harder to write, but I chose to end my life.

I wanted my time on earth to STOP.

I wanted everything to STOP.

I was tired, beyond tired.

144

Life felt completely pointless.

Quite simply, I had had enough.

I know the pain this confession brings. I know that it is so much more than words; it is an admission that I was prepared to – in fact, wanted to – leave behind this life and everything and everyone in it. I didn't want any more time, didn't want to be. I was certain that I wanted to disappear from the face of the earth and sleep forever. I no longer wanted to exist. And for those thinking rationally, those who love me, I can only begin to imagine how painful that is to hear. I can't apologise because to do so would suggest I had some level of control over this process, but I had none. I can't apologise because I did nothing wrong. It wasn't a choice, and I can now see it was a consequence of my illness, a result of my decline in mental health. And actually it wasn't only a consequence: as I saw it, it was, in fact, the cure. It was the answer I had been looking for. In the grip of my depression, I did not control my thoughts: my thoughts controlled me.

To others I might have looked like Josiah Hartley and sounded a bit like him too, but I was not him, not at that point. I was a vessel: living and making decisions with severe depression and anxiety calling all the shots. Mum had gone far away and I was glad: one less thing to think about and deal with.

It was November 2016 when I considered and then planned to die. I was nineteen years old.

Now this is strange for me because I don't know you. I know nothing about you and yet you know so much about me. And if you have been reading since the beginning you will know that this is a state of affairs that is hard for me, exposing. But as we have journeyed this far together, I would like to address you directly.

Wherever you are sitting or standing while you read this – in an office, on a bus, a beach, a sofa, the train, a plane, by a pool or in bed – I can imagine your questions and thoughts and in truth

I don't have all the answers. But I bet you are asking how I could want to disappear from the face of the earth when I had a family that loved me and so many opportunities! And I hear you, and I am grateful for your questions and your thoughts, but I can only repeat that it might have *looked* like Josiah Hartley but it was not him, not me. I was scooped out, completely hollow, and at the time it made absolute sense to cast off the pointless husk that housed my despair. I figured that by doing that I could put an end to it all, and even the thought of it was enough to bring me some small glimmer of hope, of peace.

I withdrew even further. I rarely left the mattress. I pretty much stopped eating and only sipped water, giving in to the dark cloud that threatened to consume me.

Everyone says you have to reach rock bottom before you can start to look up and move forward.

This was certainly true for me.

And this is where I was at this time.

Rock bottom.

Actually, what is beneath rock bottom? Hell? Possibly – but wherever it is, I was there and I can tell you that it was a very, very scary place.

I was both elated to have arrived somewhere, relieved in a way that I could not fall any further, and also petrified.

The worst day, the worst moment, was in fact a few days that now all blend into one dark, dark time.

There was a period of days when I lay in that quiet room and was so numb that I didn't even feel thirst.

I didn't get out of bed for days on end.

I didn't go to the loo, didn't eat, didn't drink.

I think I hoped at some level that my body would just give up, as this felt like the best thing that could happen to my head.

A cop-out, if you like, but the most attractive thought was that I would just cease to exist.

My bed was like a black hole, sucking me in. I didn't feel like part of the world. I had gone beyond feeling isolated and lonely or even sad. I felt nothing.

My life was nothing.

The future was nothing and there was nothing I could do about it, any of it.

It was a new and overwhelming sense of isolation. I tuned out the Polish chatter that filtered along the pipes and I didn't open the window or draw the curtains. The room got smaller and smaller with each passing day and I shrank with it, until I was a small coiled thing lying on the greasy sheet that sat in a lump in the middle of the mattress. My blood was thick and sluggish in my veins and my breathing slow. With my eyes closed, I drifted and I could see myself from above.

It was a pitiful sight.

I had experienced loneliness before, but this was not about being lonely. It was about feeling alone, and not just in the magnolia-painted silent walls, but alone in the world.

I felt like a dot, a floating speck in the universe, and without self-worth or importance. I could say with certainty that my death would be nothing to anyone.

I didn't matter.

Nothing mattered.

On the odd occasion when I staggered to the bathroom, I caught sight of my reflection in the mirror. It was frightening. I saw something demonised, a monster, not my true face, and that was petrifying. It only confirmed that I was right to hide away. The thought of having to go out into the outside world was unimaginable.

I was on a one-way street and it was more a case of when rather than if I would leave this life. It wasn't so much that I couldn't see a future, but more that I couldn't even see a present.

I ordered suicide pills from the Internet.

This one sentence – just seven words written so casually and yet with meaning of such magnitude.

I ordered suicide pills from the Internet.

I am deliberately keeping the name, method and details vague. But I will say that the process and purchase were staggeringly and shockingly simple. I had, I thought, managed to engineer a relatively painless death whilst leaving scope for it to be considered an accident.

And with hindsight I can see that even the smallest consideration of those left behind was a sign of hope, that all was not lost, that my life might have some value even if it was only in the eyes of those who loved me and who were going to have to say goodbye.

I remember the day the tablets arrived in the mail. They came in a silver padded pouch sitting inside a brown bubble-wrap-lined envelope, along with a pizza flyer and other junk mail, and the lot lay in a heap on the welcome mat. Having the tablets in my possession made me feel a stir of something, it gave me comfort to know that I had a way out. And all I wanted was for the nothingness, the everlasting ache of pointlessness to end. I sat on the edge of the bed and opened the pouch with its noxious contents and inhaled the scent of sulphur. They smelled as I had expected them to: dangerous, chemical-like and unpleasant. I placed the blister pack in a small gap under the washing machine, and for the first couple of days I glanced at it from time to time but after that it was enough to know that it was there. Comforting.

I wanted to pick the right time.

I wanted to disappear.

I wanted my life to stop.

Because nothing mattered . . .

I didn't say any goodbyes and I didn't write a note. In truth, neither of these things entered my mind.

It was a few days after they had arrived that I lay on the bed and stared at the gap beneath the washing machine. I could see the edge of the envelope with the tablets inside. I had no concept of the time, it could have been four in the morning or four in the afternoon, but just like that I knew it was the right time.

It was time for me to go.

I pulled the pouch from the hiding place and placed the tablets in my palm. I don't know how long I sat there looking at them, feeling the weight of them in my hand. I felt drawn to them, glad of them. They were only small, translucent with orange powder inside, and yet they were the biggest things I had ever held.

They were going to end my time.

And that was that.

I wasn't sad or overly thoughtful, just completely numb, on autopilot. I couldn't see how what came next would matter to me or to anyone. It was, like the life I had lived, inconsequential, a small thing, no more than an ending to the blip that was my existence.

Now, I don't believe in God but if divine intervention is your thing then this kind of works. I sat with my legs hanging over the side of bed, waiting for the dizziness to pass – a consequence of spending most of my time lying down and having stood up too quickly. I don't know how long I sat and waited for my head to clear, but it was long enough for fate to stick its nose in my affairs. Long enough for the universe to put me on a different path. Seconds, that was all, but seconds that made the difference.

I hadn't looked at my phone for quite a while. It was next to me on the bed and when I glanced at it it was on silent but a call was coming in. It was Simeon. I answered it almost automatically and he started with his usual jolly, 'Hey, Joshy!'

I forgot to reply, to speak; it had been a while since I had inter-
acted with anyone and after a pause he spoke again.

'Josh? Are you okay, buddy?'

I stared at the tablets in my hand and told him I was fine,
and he announced that he was in Southampton for a meeting and
would be popping in within the next half hour. I sank back on the
pillows and shoved the tablets back into the envelope. Reaching
down, I put them under my mattress. I figured it would make little
difference if I waited until tomorrow. It felt like I closed my eyes
for what I thought was no more than a minute and suddenly there
was pounding on my door.

'Hey, mate, it's Dad!' Simeon called out.

I shuffled from the bed and unlocked the door. I opened it
without considering the state of my flat, the state of me. I was
beyond that.

Simeon's face crumpled. 'Josh!'

He walked in and I watched his eyes sweep the room and his
nose wrinkle. He pulled the blinds and opened a window. The cold
air was like a sharp thing and the light hurt my eyes. I sank back
down on the mattress, weakened, and put my head on the pillow.
Simeon pushed filthy clothes, dirty plates and rubbish aside with
his foot and he sat on the floor by the side of my bed.

'It's okay, Joshy. You are going to be okay.'

I felt the unfamiliar prick of tears and gave in to the crying
that overtook me and left me breathless, taking the very last of my
energy.

Simeon sat fast. 'I am not going anywhere. I will stay here all
night. It's okay, Joshy. You just sleep now, knowing that I am right
here, mate.'

And that's what he did.

He sat on the floor, occasionally reaching out in the darkness to
hold my hand or pat my arm, uttering in a constant low murmur

that I was going to be fine . . . I was not alone . . . He was going to stay with me . . .

Some of his words permeated, others I'm sure not, but I know he stayed, just like he had when I was little and had had a bad dream, like he knew that his physical presence was enough. And it was.

I made it through the night.

When I woke the next morning, still with my thoughts hazy and my desire to leave the planet strong, Simeon was piling rubbish into bin bags and nearly gagging. I hadn't noticed how bad my surroundings had got, but it was pretty disgusting. It was a weird morning. His presence was invasive, upsetting both my plans and my routine, but at the same time I was glad he was there. We didn't chat as such; I lay down with my eyes closed, listening to him busying, and only looked up when he asked me something directly.

'You need to shower, mate.' He spoke softly, but firmly. 'And then I am taking you home.'

'I don't want—' I began.

'This isn't about what you want, Josh.' Again that tone. 'You are coming home and that's that.'

It felt nice to have someone take control. It felt like I could stop worrying, just for a bit . . .

Chapter Fifteen

AMANDA

'THE WORST KIND OF SADNESS'

'The very worst kind of sadness is the kind that doesn't have an explanation.'

Anon.

It was a bright sunny morning in my part of the world. I was sitting on a coach, travelling along in the deep forest of Queensland with a TV crew and a bunch of people when the call came in from Simeon. It was rare for him to call; the time difference made communication tricky, plus he knew that it was often difficult for me to talk freely. I was missing him and smiled as I answered the phone. When you know someone back to front and inside out, you can tell a lot about the nature of a phone call before a single word has been spoken, can accurately gauge whether it's a happy or sad call, relaxed or urgent. Simeon didn't break into the usual reassuring poetry of how much he missed me and couldn't wait to get me home. I could tell he wasn't smiling.

His pause on the other end of the phone told me that something was up and my heart raced accordingly. Had something happened to my mum or dad?

'Mandy,' he began. His rhythm was off, his tone muted.

'What's happened?' I cut to it, placing my forehead on the window as we drove the twisting lanes and roads of the rural landscape. I might have been thousands of miles away in a hot country having just done a TV show, but my heart was next to his, beating loudly with anticipation and my hand lay inside his palm.

'Joshy, erm . . .'

'Is he okay?' I tried to encourage him to get to the point; my imagination had begun to conjure unwelcome images. 'Is he okay?' I repeated, not allowing for the slightest delay on the line across the miles.

'He's home. I brought him home.'

'Oh . . .' Was that all? He was calling to tell me Josh had come home? It was odd to say the least. I waited to hear what came next and remember feeling my pulse settle because he was home and home meant safety. Simeon explained that he'd had a feeling something was off and so he pretended he had a meeting and turned up at Josh's flat.

'Righto. Well, give him my love.' I was still listening and not wanting to chat too loudly or be too open in this environment. And then came the words that made my heart race.

'He had some pills. I found them when he was in the shower. I had a look around the flat and I found some pills.'

I felt my gut churn. 'Oh, like, what kind of . . . ?' My brain was struggling to grasp what he was driving at, surely he wasn't telling me that Josh was taking drugs, surely not, was he? I mean, I *know* my kids and I knew they liked a drink, but I thought we had succeeded in warning them off drugs. 'What . . . what kind of . . . like painkillers?' I whispered.

'Pills' – and he gave me the name of them, a name I had never heard before – 'they were in a little silver padded pouch. He'd hidden them under his mattress.'

Now, the fact is I had lived with Josh for all this time and was saddened and frustrated that despite trying to crack his shell and get him to open up, I was no closer to understanding *what* had happened when he seemed to come to a mental halt right before his A levels than I was when it had *actually* happened.

It was like trying to crack an impossible puzzle and was as frustrating as it was all-consuming. My first thought was always how to make things better for him, how to help him, but my second constant nagging worry was what in the hell had happened to make my boy close down like this? And now, all this time later, Simeon was talking about pills. *Hidden* pills that he had discovered. Was that the reason for Josh's depression? Was this the answer I had been looking for?

I am ashamed to say that I felt a surge of relief, because *if* it was the case that my son was a recreational drug user and this had caused his anxiety and mental illness then at last I had something tangible I could cling to, a reason that, no matter how distasteful or hard for me to fathom, I could explore, which, hopefully, might then in turn lead to understanding and this would help me find a solution; because all I wanted to do was fix him, fix him, fix him . . .

Immediately I pictured rehabilitation centres where Josh could go and seek therapy to come off whatever noxious substance was robbing us of our boy. As usual I was running headlong into solution mode without asking enough questions. I started to think of people who might have more experience in this field than me, people I could ask about the best course of action, this before I even knew what drug it was my son was addicted to.

But of course, you, dear readers, are a few steps ahead of me at this point. You know that Josh was not addicted to drugs, as did my husband. Simeon is an army officer and is very drug aware, he has to be because of the army's zero tolerance policy towards drugs and he feels a strong commitment to the pastoral care and health of his recruits. He knew what he had found. I heard him draw a deep breath and what he said next threw me. His words landed like a punch to the side of my head.

'They were suicide pills, Mandy. He was in a really bad way.'

I tried to speak, but my voice had withered away and my throat had closed. My limbs shook and I thought I might be sick. I closed my eyes and pushed my head harder against the window, trying to blot out the background noise and chatter on the coach.

I would be lying if I said I had never thought about *how* he might do it *if* he chose to do it. Would it be by noose, exhaust pipe, blade? Which would be the tool or method by which my son would come undone? And now I knew because Simeon had found his pills.

'I don't understand. What? How? Where are you? Where is he? What's happening?' I croaked.

'It's all fine. He's fine. It's okay, Mandy . . .'

But I knew it was not okay. Nothing was okay. And his words irritated me. I remember him telling me to stay calm over and over – 'try and stay calm' – and that 'it was all going to be okay', which I knew by this point was a lie. I know I cried while my mind raced and my tongue simultaneously struggled to catch up. 'So did he, had he, I mean, is he okay?' I felt my voice crack. Simeon has since told me that all I did was keep asking is he okay? Where is he now? And again: is he okay? As if his words of reassurance would not sink in or I just wasn't listening. I remember hearing my husband's slow intake of breath – whether he was tired or crying, I couldn't tell. 'He's sleeping,' he managed, and this fact did calm me down, because if my son was sleeping and Simeon was watching over him then I knew for the time being at least, he was safe. I could then clearly tell that Simeon was crying and I matched him tear for tear. And that was how we sat on the other side of the world from each other, the silence punctuated only by our tears.

I shan't ever forget it.

We arranged to speak later, and I sat very still, waiting for the world to stop spinning and I sobbed, quietly. The atmosphere on the bus was party-like. People were chatting and laughing loudly, recounting the morning we had spent and making plans for later. I felt quite removed from the whole thing.

Now, it's a funny thing in life how in certain situations you discover that the kindness of strangers can make all the difference. It's like the universe sends you a guardian angel to get you through. I might have been crying more noisily than I thought, I don't know, but what I do know is that what happened next was something quite pivotal in both Josh's and my recovery, certainly in how I perceived his illness.

I looked up and the man sitting in front had put his hand in the gap between the seats. He and I had been on this crazy Australian adventure together, both part of a larger group, and I had always found him very funny, extremely kind and refreshingly outspoken. He was sitting next to his girlfriend, also a beautiful soul, and when his hand appeared it felt like the most natural thing in the world to hold it.

'Are you okay?' he asked.

I told him in so many words that my son had depression. And that by the sounds of things he had tried to take his own life. It was a bizarre thing to be saying, bizarre and unimaginable, and yet it also felt good to be able to talk to someone, this relative stranger, about it. He told me it was good that Josh was not on his own.

He spoke softly, sharing with me a personal story of someone close to him who had found themselves in a similar situation. He then offered me some advice, small words given without any fanfare. I wonder if he will even remember the incident or what he said to me, but his words have stayed with me and are ones I consider even today when the going gets tough and I find myself at a loss, heading, as I often do, straight into solution mode, sometimes even when there is no solution to be found.

He said, 'You know this is nothing to do with you, don't you?' That was it. That was all.

I smiled, brightened a little and said, 'Thank you. Yes, I know it's probably not because of something I did wrong or did or didn't do.'

'No.' He shook his head and smiled. I had clearly misunderstood. 'I mean it is *nothing to do with you*. This is Josh's journey, Josh's battle, and he will have to figure it out. You can't do it for him.'

It was a light-bulb moment, but not the one I had hoped for. My dreams of seeing the answer to Josh's problems spelled out for me to read and act upon were dashed. It was a terrible day: the thought, the *idea*, that the person I love most in the whole wide world would rather not be here on this planet is one of the most difficult things I have ever had to try to get to grips with. My thoughts instantly, painfully and narcissistically leapt to the idea that I *had* done something wrong, that I had been a bad mother, that I could and should have done things differently.

The lovely man on the coach was right, of course he was right. And it was a moment of clarity that eased my burden and made me think about how I was going to act going forward. I got what he was telling me: that Josh had to understand what was happening to him. Josh had to try to solve the puzzle of his mental health and only when he understood the puzzle and could make sense of the maze in which he was lost, he might just, if we were lucky, be able to find a way out.

His calm, clear expression, spoken with insight and devoid of emotion, got me through the trip. I am thankful for the kindness of that stranger every day.

The coach arrived back at the fancy hotel we were staying in and I rushed to my room, desperate to speak to Simeon. I sat on the wide, soft bed in the beautiful bedroom and wanted nothing more than to be at home.

With the phone held tight, Simeon told me that Josh didn't know it but he had taken the tablets from his room.

'He doesn't know I have them. I think it was close, Mand, I got there and . . . Don't cry, darling. Don't cry . . .'

He gave me only the most rudimentary of details as to the state Josh had been in when he got to him, keeping the true horror of his situation for when I got home, knowing it was far better that he be there to gather me up when I fell.

He described the silver pouch and we both wondered about the faceless person or organisation who packed, taped and stamped these parcels of death and distributed them in exchange for money to desperate, needy, hurt or damaged people all over the world.

People like our son.

It was like a punch in the gut to think of how close we might have come to losing Josh. This was real. Simeon told me they were small, translucent gel capsules that could easily have been mistaken for a chemist-bought cure for aches and pains; these were the tiny tablets that had the power to send our boy to sleep and take him away from us forever. I wanted to howl my sadness but I was unable. Instead, the gush of tears rendered me silent and I sank down on to the bed, coiled and shaking, as my husband tried to reassure me from the other side of the world, whispering all the platitudes I too would have spoken if it had been his distress that poured down the line, his throat raw with desperation and his breath faltering.

'The good thing is I found them, Mandy.'

'If he'd wanted to take them, he would have done so immediately.'

'We can talk to him about it when the time is right.'

'He's still here, Mandy. He is still here!'
'I won't let him out of my sight . . .'

I was and am always grateful for his words, but couldn't shake the thought that yes, we could get rid of these, but what was to stop Josh buying more?

I felt hopeless, beaten and oh so far away.

It was one of my lowest days, for sure.

There I was staying in a luxury hotel involved in an amazing project with some brilliant people, some of whom are still my great friends to this day. I was trying to be bright and up and yet Simeon's discovery, proof that suicide had been, even if only fleeting, our boy's intention, made me ask the same question over and over: why am I here? What the hell am I doing? I could only picture my fractured little family and my gut ached with the desire to get back to them.

I decided to keep the terrible facts to myself and not bring everyone around me down and so I did my very best to paint on a smile and join in, counting down the hours, minutes and seconds until I got home, which was about five days from when I took the phone call. I desperately wanted to see Josh, knowing my mind would not settle until I had seen his face and I was also ridiculously fearful that Simeon might not be giving me the full story – was Josh hurt? Damaged? And the answer to that was yes, yes he was. He didn't want to speak to me on the phone and I now know he didn't want to talk to anyone – he simply took to his bed and closed down, sleeping.

I have never been so relieved to feel a plane touch down in my whole life. Having left Josh at home with my parents in the house, Simeon met me at arrivals and we spent the drive home going over every aspect of what had happened to Josh during my absence. Simeon looked absolutely exhausted and drawn, and he explained that he had been watching over Josh, literally, since he had bundled him into the car. He explained how they ate a little together, mainly soup, and how he had run Josh baths and made sure he had a glass of water. The basics. I sat quietly and it was like listening to an audio play – one where you are gripped and stunned into silence because the words are so powerful and disturbing, and all you can do is feel thankful that it's not real and that it's not anyone you love being discussed . . . But it *was* real and it was Josh we were discussing. I was actually too numb to cry. Simeon described the absolute squalor that Josh's lovely flat had fallen into, the smell of a body unwashed, living among dirt. He told me how he had slept on the floor of Josh's bedroom so he was not alone in the darkness, but worse than this was the way he described Josh's expression.

'It's like he's there, but not there . . . His eyes are empty.'

'Where's he gone, Simeon?' I whispered.

He could only shake his head; neither of us had the answer to that one.

I felt terrible that Simeon had been coping with this alone while I was away. I felt sick. We have discussed it since and he says that ironically it was probably better that I was away. In my absence he felt able to take complete control without intervention or hesitation and also that my sometimes overly emotional responses helped no one, especially Josh. But this did not stop the flare of jealousy in my gut that in Josh's darkest hour it had been Simeon who had come to the rescue, Simeon who Josh had leaned on – that had always been my job! But I kept this to myself. Despite my utter bewilderment and shock at what had happened I knew enough to keep schtum about some misplaced envy when all my husband deserved was my eternal gratitude. But that's how it was.

We talked about how we should handle things going forward, Simeon reminding me that I had to try to hold it together and that we needed to keep the atmosphere as calm as we could, the best it could be, to allow Josh peace and rest, to allow recovery at his own pace.

'We need help, Sim. Josh needs help – professional help – even if he says he doesn't or refuses, we need to do what we think is right for him.'

'Yep.'

We were in agreement, although where and how we were to find that help was a daunting prospect.

We decided not to mention the discovery of the pills to Josh for the time being. It was very clear that our boy was in a bad place and we agreed that any forced discussion on such a sensitive subject, any pressure, negativity or perceived judgement adding to a mind already teetering on the edge, was not a good thing. It was a wonderful relief to walk into our little house and see him, a little pale with dark circles under his haunted eyes, a little jumpy, but present, alive and present.

I felt an overwhelming desire to run to him, wrap my arms around him and collapse – the very opposite of what Simeon and I had agreed Josh needed, and so I checked myself and managed to keep it together – just.

Over the next few days and weeks we, as a family, hunkered down and pulled up the drawbridge, dedicating ourselves to being present for Josh, organising an informal rota that meant that one of us was always in the house, within reach and keeping an eye. Mum and Dad knew what had happened and we told Ben. All bore the same stunned expression as I had when I heard; it was and still is a shocking thing to consider. We literally watched him for twenty-four hours a day, waking at the slightest sound in the middle of the night, taking it in turns to stand over Josh and stare at his face screwed up in a tortured sleep, restoring his covers, bringing him water.

I remember telling a friend I was going to miss their party – my excuse was probably flimsy and I don't think they have spoken to me since! I couldn't even begin to explain how irrelevant a party or socialising felt when we were dealing with something so all-consuming and scary. It's at times like this you truly find out who your real friends are. The moment I stepped inside the house the weight of what we were living with pushed down on my shoulders until it felt almost impossible to move.

I remembered my fellow traveller's words on the coach and tried to create a neutral atmosphere where Josh could just 'be', where he could figure things out. For the next few weeks or so, I would place his supper in front of him and say 'hello' as he sloped into the kitchen to get a glass of water or smile as I passed him on the stairs. Trying to conjure an air of normality was very close to torture. I was screaming on the inside, *We found your pills! Where did you get them? Why did you buy them? Talk to me, Josh! Talk to someone! We are here for you! We love you! Please don't leave us! It will get better! It will! Please, please, please, Josh, don't leave us! Don't do that, don't ever do that! We love you! We all love you so much!*

This last phrase – *we love you!* – I realised I had been using as a cure-all his whole life. It is only now as we begin to come out the other side that I understand how meaningless and insignificant this phrase is to someone who doesn't feel any love in the world, who feels nothing at all and who believes that to opt out of life might be the best thing.

Josh looked and acted like a wild thing caged. Eye contact was minimal, his body and face twitched and his bedroom was a tip. Clothes were all over the floor as well as general rubbish, empty drink cans, food-encrusted plates. He had taken root in his room and I understood that. The small space in the corner of our little house was his refuge, his haven, and if he wanted to live in it undisturbed, then who was I to intervene? I didn't like the chaos of his environment, but felt it was important that when his life was spiralling faster than he could cling on, any element of control that I could give him was important.

You don't want to wash? Fine.

You don't want me to clean your room? Okay.

You want to eat alone under the duvet? All right then.

I was tormented with a particular set of thoughts before I fell asleep each night. I pictured Josh as a baby and a small child when he would place his chubby hand in mine and smile at me because I was the person who knew how to make everything feel a little bit better. And yet the fact was I hadn't been there when he needed me the most. I couldn't think about it without feeling the room spin and having to push my feet into the floor just to know that *I* was on solid ground.

The thought that I was on the other side of the world in his moment of need fills me with sadness topped with a froth of guilt. I can only begin to imagine what this might have felt like had he succeeded, had it been his last day on earth.

The myriad of people I have met from all walks of life who have lost a child, a lover, a friend, a partner, a parent, a sibling – a life taken by their own hand – they show a level of resilience and strength which I envy and admire and suspect I would not possess.

I spoke to one woman who told me that she would never, ever get over it, but that 'life goes on, what else can you do?'

I think about her words a lot, *what else can you do?* She and all others with whom I have discussed their loss share sentiments that echo with self-recrimination.

Why didn't I check on him?
Why didn't I call her that morning?
How could he choose to leave us?
What signs did I miss?
What could I have done differently?
Was it my fault?

These sentiments are as futile as they are heartbreaking. The pain of those left behind is unimaginable to me.

I asked Josh in more recent times what was going through his mind when he wanted to die. His reply was both simple and complex, jarring and strangely reassuring. 'I felt a little elated, relieved that the exhaustion was going to stop. I had my ending all figured out. I felt peaceful for the first time in as long as I could remember. I felt the pressure lift a little from my shoulders and my mind cleared, like fog being sucked from a room. I guess a bit like I was tired, no, beyond tired, absolutely bone-breakingly exhausted, and someone had put a hand on my shoulder and said, "You can go to sleep now. It's okay, Josh, you can go to sleep . . ."'

And weirdly, I took comfort from this – the idea that had the unimaginable happened, this would have been his last thought, one of peace, calm and, dare I say, something close to happiness. I am of course *fully* aware that I have the luxury of being able to ask Josh these questions, something painfully denied to all those who have over the years shared their stories with me.

The one thing I have to remind myself of on days when the fear feels a little overwhelming is that no matter how bad it is for me it is a million times worse for Josh. And again I think of the wise advice I was given: this is Josh's journey and I am but a bystander who can only do what I can, and that sometimes feels like very little. That one brief phone call received on a coach on the other side of the world meant I went from being a mum who viewed her son's life in terms of next year . . . next decade . . . to looking at it in terms of twenty-four hours . . .

Even now, over three years later, when I arrive home I put the key in the door and call out loudly 'Hello, darling? All okay?', only feeling my pulse settle when I have heard him call out in return.

Can you imagine that? Every single time I arrive home, and once I have heard his voice, I breathe deeply, knowing that today is a good one because he is still here. My beautiful boy has made it another day.

Chapter Sixteen

Josh

'It's not my fault!'

'Doctors put drugs of which they know little into bodies of which they know less for diseases of which they know nothing at all.'

Voltaire

I actually remember very little about the time immediately after I returned home from Southampton. It's foggy. I know I was in a pretty bad way and took to my bed, literally only venturing out when I had to. I was vaguely aware of Mum and Simeon watching me. Constantly watching me, which drove me crazy. My horizontal life spent on a mattress was so normal for me that I was always slightly surprised by the way others got out of bed, had a shower, put clothes on and went outside into the world where they would interact with other people. This only added to my sense of isolation. Why could they do it and I couldn't? I was no more capable of that, any of it, than flying to the moon.

Mum and Simeon continued to look at me warily; their fear came off them in waves and if anything it made *me* feel even more afraid. Because these were the people who were supposed to be in control and if they were worried and fearful, then, fuck me, it wasn't a ride I wanted to be on. There were more lucid moments when I felt pissed off that I had been prevented from following the course of action I had decided upon. Pissed off that they hadn't left me alone. I pictured the pills I'd stashed under the mattress in my studio flat and wasn't that fussed, knowing I could easily get more – they were locked in my room and I had the only key, I didn't think they would be discovered.

My life was reduced to no more than my immediate needs. Going to the loo, eating a bit, drinking water . . . that was about it. I developed acute anxiety about opening emails and taking phone calls. I can't explain why, but it felt that whatever might be waiting for me inside any message would only be bad and I had to avoid them at all costs. This I easily solved by never checking my emails and keeping my phone switched off – simple. Nan and Grandad visited and looked at me with bewildered expressions of love. I knew they wanted to make me feel better and were eaten up by not being able to help. I hate that I put them through that. I heard Ben's voice on the landing and he put his head around the door on his way in or out.

'Hey.'

'Hey.'

I lived a half-life.

It was no life – and I thought it would never end.

Mum and Simeon kept suggesting that I needed to talk to a professional but I refused point blank. I can't fully explain why – maybe I didn't want to have it confirmed how bad things were and maybe I didn't want Mum and Simeon to have it confirmed how bad things were and – as far as I was aware – they did not know of my intention to end my life. I think it was from a combination of my growing desperation and their exasperation that eventually I reluctantly agreed to go and visit our GP.

I know that as I climbed into the car, Mum said, 'Do you want to get changed, Josh?'

I looked down at my sweatpants with food stuck to them and my less-than-pristine T-shirt. My hair I knew was greasy, but what I could not begin to figure out was why it mattered. I shrugged and off we went.

At some level I had high hopes of medical intervention. I was physically and mentally weary. Sick and tired of feeling so low, I wanted an instant fix, a cure. I wanted that feeling when you open your eyes on the penultimate day of flu, right before the 'completely better' day, and the fug of illness has started to lift, and the world looks a bit brighter, hunger rumbles, replacing the cavernous void that has sat in your gut. You can breathe easier, the thought of a bath does not make you cry, and your head stops spinning, your limbs are lighter and you lift your head from the dent in the pillow and realise that there is more to the world than the four walls inside of which you are cloistered. Of course I wanted this – who wouldn't? And I mean, how hard could it be? This is the twenty-first century; we transplant organs to give a new lease of life and we are giving HIV a good kicking! Heck, even a cancer diagnosis is no longer a death sentence and we can fertilise eggs outside of the human body and transplant them into a host, creating life for couples where nature needs a helping hand. I therefore assumed that with the number of people suffering with depression spiralling in all walks of life, surely, surely there would be a pill I could take? A medicine I could swallow? A patch to adhere to my skin? An exercise to alleviate my symptoms? A bloody cure?

Apparently not.

I sat in front of the GP and heard her heavy sigh in response to my question as to what kind of help was available and what did she recommend? I must admit my hopes were not as high after I had, for the last couple of minutes, listened to her ask me the most surface-level questions, as if I had walked in with a head cold or an ankle sprain. She made me feel like just another number walking through the door and seemed uninterested.

'It's not quite that simple,' was her opening line.

I could have guessed . . .

'We can start you on some medication and see how it goes?' she offered quickly and without conviction, doing little to give me any faith in the drug she wanted me to pump into my system. I wasn't even made aware of what the drug was or how it worked. And I had hoped for something with more certainty. Before I had a chance to answer or ask questions, she began tip-tapping into her keyboard, as if the decision had been made and I wondered what I had missed – was that it? No discussion, no referral? Nothing. I had been in the room for mere minutes and here we were with her signing her name to a prescription and me realising that this was all that was on offer. Take it or leave it. But this was, after all, what I wanted, wasn't it?

The decision to go down the antidepressant route was not one I took lightly. I am ashamed to admit that back then I viewed those who took prescription meds for the condition in a less than favourable way. I guess I thought they might have taken the easy route and had fallen for the promise of a cure. But as I sat in that chair I laughed, realising that despite my pre-conceived ideas, despite the lack of a guarantee, I wanted that cure too, and who could blame me for that? I had wanted to believe there was another way. A better way. I guess I have never liked the idea of being drug-dependent, didn't want to consume something daily that would mess with my brain, but even I had to admit, my brain was already messed with, so what did I have to lose?

If I had to picture someone regularly taking antidepressants, I saw the image of a person spaced out, unable to function or climb out of bed without reaching for their drug of choice, but by this stage I was desperate and desperation is a powerful motivator. I would have done anything and taken anything recommended to me if I had thought for a second that it might make my suffering end. Plus the reality was I was *already* spaced out, unable to function or climb out of bed. What was the worst that could happen?

The trouble was I had been raised in a house where tablets and medicine were often the last thing to reach for when illness struck, rather than the first. In our house, a headache was cured with a big glass of water, some fresh air and a nap. Colds with hot water, honey and lemon . . . You get the idea. So to reach for tablets, to cash in the paper slips that both of the healthcare professionals I had visited waved under my nose felt like a big deal.

I had briefly in the preceding weeks discussed the possibility of taking a course of antidepressants with my parents and the thing that struck me was how readily they had agreed.

'Why not?'

'You need to try lots of things.'

'They might help . . .'

'Lots of people take them.'

I knew then how desperate they were to help find my cure. Mum did not once mention an organic alternative and Simeon's expression was almost pleading.

And there I was sitting in front of the GP who was typing out a prescription for a drug called Citalopram. It felt almost inevitable that I would start to put this substance into my system and once I had accepted the thought, I then allowed myself to feel a small level of optimism – could this really make me feel . . . make me *feel*?

Citalopram – a strange-sounding drug of which I was instructed to take 15mg once a day. The GP signed the prescription with a flourish and I took it next door to the pharmacy – feeling a little grubby and a little hopeful. The box with a blister pack strip resting inside made a pleasing rattle in the palm of my hand. It was literally something to cling to, a man-made cure, I hoped. It was the first thing I was doing that was proactive in trying to get better – an attempt to be well.

Mum was chirpy back in the car – if my optimism was at one per cent hers was a hundred. Bloody typical, she was completely unaware of her irritation factor or the added pressure this put on me – I *had* to get better. This *had* to work.

I took one of the tablets as soon as I got home, swallowing it with a glass of water, keen to get the regimen started. Once I had taken it, all worries over the contents and side effects of the drug went out of the window. That was it, I was on board. I went back to my bed and waited.

I remember Mum smiling at me over the table as I swallowed the pill, as if to say 'well?' and I wanted to tell her to fuck off! What did she think? One hit and I'd be restored? Fine? Returned? I reminded her that it would take at least two weeks before I saw or felt any possible change.

And in fact this turned out to be true.

There *was* a change after two weeks, but it was not the change I had been hoping for. Not the change any of us had been hoping for. Like anything that happens gradually it's only when the effects are at their strongest that you fully appreciate a change. I became aware that my thoughts were foggier, if that was possible, and I was out of sorts, confused. I was also disappointed that my mood had not picked up and my energy levels were still so low. I went back to the same GP after two weeks, as instructed, and there was very little discussion about my actual symptoms, which I outlined. It was hard to explain in my present state that I had felt foggy before but now I was foggier, I'd been tired but now I was more tired, but it was the truth. Her immediate suggestion was to up my dosage to 30mg a day, this after just two weeks. I went home and immediately took 30mg – double the previous amount. Within days I felt itchy, like my skin was crawling, but was unsure if the itchiness was connected to the Citalopram and so I carried on taking it, wanting to feel the positive effects of the increased dose. Eventually Mum called the GP and she was told that it would be the standard two weeks for my body to settle into the new drug and stabilise and that the itchiness would probably stop.

A day or so later and my reaction to the increased dosage was so severe that I was feeling very sick, physically ill as well as mentally. It was a new low for me. I was used to not being able to think straight but now? It was not only my standard joint pain that bothered me, but I was covered in angry hives, a severe allergic reaction that occurred all over my hips, back, bum, chest, arms and legs. It was horrific. I was sore and my mental decline continued until I was so foggy and drunk-feeling that I wobbled physically, nearly falling over. I felt fearful and I could not stop crying. This overly emotional state was a new one on me. On the few occasions over the past few months when I had managed to cry it had been a welcome release of sorts. This was nothing like that. There was no upside, just pure distress.

I remember standing in the kitchen in my pyjamas with tears pouring down my face, embarrassed, distressed and hollow. It was awful to see the faces of those around me, my nan and grandad especially, who I knew were watching closely, knowing I was now taking tablets to make me better. They would look into my eyes searching for the old Josh – and as I lumbered into the room and grazed the wall, crying with my face bloated, skin sore and my head pounding, their distress was apparent. This reaction from them was only marginally easier to handle than their usual false smiles and questions of, 'Are they working yet, darling? Are you feeling any better?'

◆ ◆ ◆

The hives settled a little, but my lethargy and sadness did not. Mum decided to book an appointment with a psychiatrist – this in part as a result of the lack of engagement from our GP – but progress was painfully slow. A Royal College of Psychiatrists' survey of the experience of 500 diagnosed mental health patients found that some had waited up to thirteen years to get the treatment they needed.[12] A quarter of the 500 patients, who were drawn from across the UK, waited more than three months to see an NHS mental health specialist. Six per cent had waited at least a year.

I think it's fair to say I was slipping. I could have lived with the side effects had the drugs positively affected my mood, but the uplift was so negligible it wasn't worth it. I railed against seeing a psychiatrist. I did not want to go down that route, did not want to come away feeling the same level of disappointment I had felt with both the previous therapist and the GPs I had seen. The very word psychiatrist filled me with dread; that was where you were shown ink splats and asked for your thoughts, right? It was for people who were nuts, wasn't it? Was that me? Was I actually losing my mind? The thought was petrifying. I was of course aware that psychiatrists were different from therapists in that they were qualified doctors who could hand out prescriptions. But regardless, I did not want to go.

I felt pressure from Mandy and Simeon to do something and thought that if I went once to see a psychiatrist it might at least get them off my back.

It turned out, however, to be one of the most positive encounters I had – I liked him. He was smart. We had a connection and there was not an ink splat in sight. Unlike with the GP, I didn't feel like he was watching the clock to hurry me back out of the door. I didn't know what to expect from psychiatry, didn't know how it would be of benefit, but I honestly wish I had gone to see him sooner. He sat behind a desk and it felt more business-like than medical and that suited me. He was interested in my studies and spoke to me calmly like an equal. I trusted him; I guess that was the fundamental difference.

He too asked me if there was any one thing that had happened, one traumatic event? One memory that scarred, something on which I could hang my illness, but again all I could do was shake my head and tell him that no, there was nothing . . .

He then said: 'I bet you kind of wish there was because as *terrible* as that would be at least you and everyone else could understand it, relate to it. It would be a starting point.'

'Exactly.' He got it.

He asked me about my medical history, my family history, explaining things to me on a biological level, to which I responded well. He then told me something that was simple and yet radical. It has stayed with me. It was the first time it had been said expressly and it altered the way I viewed my illness, he said: 'You know this isn't your fault, Josh, don't you?'

I stared at him, a little overcome with emotion.

I nodded, only half believing him, despite our very factual discussion.

'Seriously, Josh' – he spoke more earnestly now, leaning forward to hold my eyeline – 'you have an illness and it is not your fault. Just like if you had a physical illness, cancer or whatever, you wouldn't blame yourself then, would you?'

I shook my head again.

'Well, this is no different. You have an illness. You have severe depression. An illness. And just like any illness you need to be kind to yourself and give yourself time to heal and we can give you drugs that can help with that process. Okay?'

'Okay.' I cried again.

Now, it might sound odd, but until he said this to me, it did not fully occur to me that I was ill. I knew things weren't right, but I thought I was weak, going through a blip, a crisis, crazy . . . call it what you like, but ill? My God, that was it, I was ill!

His words were like scissors cutting me free of some of the ties that bound me to my depression. I can now see that this was the start of what led to my recovery. A small beginning, like cracking open the window in a previously airless room, like shining a thin beam of light into a dark chamber, like removing a plug from my ear to allow the smallest sound to filter in where before there had only been silence. I can see his mouth forming the words, hear his voice sounding them and I realised that it was not my fault . . . *It was not my fault . . . It was not my fault . . .*

He explained that there was an almost infinite range of drugs with an almost infinite combination of dosages and it was about trying them out until we found the make and dose that was right for me. This information was more than deflating; it felt like I still had a mountain to climb before I was going to get the medicine that might make a difference.

He noted my crestfallen expression and said, 'I am going to write you a new prescription and the good news, Josh, is that if this doesn't work there is another make to try and another one and another one.'

I smiled, despite feeling gutted, even after everything I still hoped I might be able to take one magic tablet that would make it all disappear.

The next drug was called Mirtazapine. I knew the drill by now and went straight to the pharmacy. I was to take half a pill, 15mg, for a few days and then up the dose to a full 30mg. The effects of Mirtazapine came on a lot, lot quicker.

I was aware of feeling very foggy and of a new drunk sensation. My speech was impaired, garbled and most crucially I slept for up to eighteen hours a day, after which I would reluctantly wake and eat to feed the huge increase in my appetite. I quickly gained weight and my face was bloated, eyes sunken. I couldn't stand to see my reflection and it was during this time that my self-loathing was at its height, which only fuelled my depression. I didn't feel like part of the human race. I was detached from society like a strange creature that spends its life sleeping, eating, battling nightmares, repeat . . .

This was how I lived for six months.

It was terrible, really terrible. I can't even stand to think about it. It wasn't living.

Chapter Seventeen

Amanda

'The boy with all the gifts'

'There is a comfort in the strength of love; 'Twill make
a thing endurable, which else would overset the brain,
or break the heart.'

William Wordsworth

Josh was on his second brand of medication, the effects of which
were devastating. He was bloated and almost catatonic at times,
only stirring to eat and then falling asleep again. They seemed toxic
to him. I researched their effects and the message seemed to be the
same – that it would take time, time for his body to adjust, time
for them to do their job. He persevered. And we watched – at a
loss as to what else to try and grateful for the fact that he was willing to try them, try something. I kept hoping, praying that they
would start doing what they promised and make him feel better. If
not completely better then at least better long enough to give him
some respite from his depression, a break from the debilitating

fatigue. I figured this rest would help with his exhaustion and this in turn would allow for healing. Whilst I was wary of him becoming dependent on antidepressants, by the time we *finally* managed to get him to a GP I was willing to try anything, literally anything that might help him; we were determined to do all we could to stop Josh from trying to take his own life.

By this stage it was apparent to anyone who came into our home that Josh was very poorly. I remember the looks on the faces of countless visitors when Josh would appear, in his PJs, his hair hanging over his face, unspeaking and glancing in their direction, eyes averted, as if trying to figure out whether he knew the person and what was expected of him. It broke my heart. I would then rush in with a smile and cheery, 'Oh, Joshy is not too great today, why don't you go back to bed, darling? Can I bring you anything?' wanting to put him out of the misery of the interaction.

Whilst we didn't trumpet the situation to all and sundry, we were open with family and friends and anyone who asked – about the fact that he was suffering with severe depression. I had at first shied away from the admission, still in the back of my mind hoping that the old adage of 'least said soonest mended' might apply and that he would bounce back without the stigma of mental illness trailing him for life. And then something quite surprising happened and it was something I had not banked on, but with the admission to others that Josh had depression came a wide and varied range of reactions. Some were kind, humbling, supportive and others downright fury-inducing, ignorant and unkind.

You see here's the thing: my son was born with all the gifts. He was born without disability in a shiny hospital where medical equipment and medicine were freely available, and that hospital was situated in a wealthy country free from war, famine and the dangers of extreme weather. He was born to a family who loved and nurtured him. He had a home, a permanent and pleasant roof over his head. He was supported, educated and cared for, so what the hell did he have to be depressed about, right?

WRONG! WRONG! WRONG!

THIS was very often the question I was asked:

'What does *he* have to be depressed about?'

'*Depressed?* Why is *he* depressed?'

'*Josh?* Depressed? How does that work?'

'*He just needs to get a job.*'

I could go on . . . These are just some of the subtle variants of the questions I have been asked over the years, but all with the same slant, the same angle, the same underlying message. And it's a message commonly configured in the thoughts of the ignorant and the ill-informed, the sneerers, the disbelievers and the jolly, confident authorities on the subject who have *never* experienced anything like the sinister sickness that is depression. It made me angry then and it makes me so very angry now!

What they were actually saying with that question was:

'*How can someone with all the gifts be depressed? It makes no sense; he just needs to pull himself together. I mean he looks okay . . . Is he just lazy? There are hungry people begging on the streets right now and Josh is not one of them! I don't get it! There are people fighting wars while he's at home with a remote control for the TV within reach! There are people who have lost their homes . . . been injured in a fire . . . coping with loss . . . struggling with debt . . . I have had worse and I am not depressed!*'

I then have to fight the urge to yell, '*Well bloody good for you!*'

On and on it goes. I can assure you that the list of all the people and all the situations in the whole wide world who are much, much, much worse off than Josh is a long one. And yet here we are!

And to all those people who knit their brows, tighten their lips and pull their heads back on their shoulders in judgement, I would say this:

Imagine if you turned from the stove where your attention was on making brunch and someone you dearly loved was sitting at the table crying, sobbing with a terribly broken arm. I am not talking a bit broken, but shattered, lacerated, crushed, mangled, hanging limp and useless and you took them to a doctor, who said, 'Well, I'm not sure what to do to make it better. There are several things we *could* try that *might* work . . . but then again they might not.'

And so you carefully, so very carefully help them back into the car and call their place of work/place of study to explain that this terrible thing has befallen them. Now imagine the person on the end of the line hums a little to let you know that they hope it's *not* going to be a long-term thing because long-term things are irritating, inconvenient and costly and it is in fact far, far better for everyone that we get 'Back on track ASAP!'

And meanwhile the person you love is still sobbing, 'Please make it stop! It hurts so badly! Make it stop! Help me!'

And you dance around in a state of panic because you don't know *how* to help them! You pull out your hair, trying to figure out what to do! But you are not trained. And you are scared. How do you heal their pain, make everything better? How do you help them live a life while the broken bones dangle and fingers start falling off and the skin is raw . . .

'Please make it stop! It hurts! Please! I can't stand it much longer!' they scream louder and louder and your gut folds in response, partly because of their pain but also your inability to fix it.

And then you draw on all your courage and decide you need to ask for help, because you can't do it alone and you think the best thing is to tell family, friends and neighbours that the reason your loved one has been a little out of sorts, and you have gone MIA (unable to attend parties or meet for coffee or go to the cinema or for a walk), is because this terrible, unwanted thing has happened to them, and they need support and understanding, as do you, because it has made

179

you boring, the very opposite of a fun person to spend time with. You gently explain their arm has become *destroyed* and the affliction is unrelentingly painful and useless, a liability! They can't rest, can't work, can't sleep, can't even think straight! And trying to figure out how to fix it is not easy or quick and maybe not even possible. This mangled, painful state of affairs might, in fact, be as good as it gets.

And now imagine the person you have taken into your confidence, this family/friend/neighbour to whom you have courageously revealed the extent of your loved one's injury, their pain – imagine that their response is this:

'Oh, my friend had that, but she's fine now. She did yoga and drank healing tea. I think my brother had it too. He became a vegan and took up scuba diving.'

And you stare mystified and utter, 'Thank you. I might suggest that.'

But they are not done.

'Have they tried *using* the arm? Couldn't they just pick up a box? Try it out? Get out of bed? And pick up a box?'

('Why doesn't Josh just go for a walk, just a little stroll? Fresh air does wonders!')

And you reply, with a smile at first, 'Well, no. They can't use the arm. It's hanging off, the bones are broken, the skin raw, it's a mess . . . they are in pain.'

('Josh can't get out of bed. He can't stay awake . . .')

'Well, I'm not suggesting a *big* box, but what about a small box to start with and then who knows . . .'

This time you answer a little more firmly, 'Well, no. Their arm doesn't work, not at all and it affects the other arm, in fact it affects everything. They are in pain, they are bed-bound, they are overwhelmed and exhausted from living like this.'

('His brain is broken and he can't think about anything else, can't think at all . . .')

'What about a teeny tiny little box?'

And you have to bite your tongue and resist the temptation of picking up the metaphorical box and shoving it up their metaphorical arse because they just don't get it!

When something is broken, by definition it doesn't work! And depression is a brain that is broken. It is an illness. A fracture. A sickness. A malaise. And no one, no one on the face of the earth, no matter where or how they are born or what gifts they are born with or without, would choose to be depressed. Got it?

GOOD.

Now imagine trying to have that conversation as the sufferer, where you are in pain, worn down, exhausted by your illness and on top of this you have to overcome the prejudice, the assumed knowledge and the misconceptions. This was certainly my experience. I remember one acquaintance I had confided in saying to me, 'God, everyone's depressed. Think I'd quite like it, a week in bed with someone bringing me tea, I could do with that!' I was speechless, could only picture Josh's face like that of an old man, moving around his mattress with restless boredom, fatigue and a mind that just would not stop whirring at 3 a.m. and I felt my tears pool.

And *this* before we even touch on the stigma and the fear that mental illness is at best unpredictable and at worst, contagious! Yes, really, some people don't want to catch it. I am rolling my eyes now and putting down my laptop to go in search of tea, healing tea, I hope. I need to calm down . . .

◆ ◆ ◆

Okay, two cups drunk and it has helped, a little.

I came to think of Josh's depression as a dark monster, a shadow that lived under our roof. A huge monster of which we were all afraid. A subject so frightening we thought it best, at times, not to mention it. And as if that wasn't bad enough we all pretended we couldn't see the monster!

Can you imagine? Walking cautiously around, taking part in the most horrible of pantomimes. Tiptoeing around Josh, masquerading that all was well, chatting about the day ahead while passing the milk over the breakfast table for the cornflakes with the radio playing in the background, while Josh sat in the chair opposite and cried.

'He's behind you!'

And yes, he was behind us; he was at the table when we ate, looking over our shoulder while we cleaned our teeth at night and he even sat at the bottom of the bed, staring at me while I made my twice-nightly visit to the bathroom. Once to use the loo, the second time, an hour later, simply to add variation, a change of scenery in the tumultuous wee small hours when the house was cold and the mountain we had to climb felt insurmountable and I couldn't stop my cogs from turning. It was rare for me to sleep through the night, and if I woke in the early hours that would be it, no going back to sleep. I found the world to be the loneliest and quietest at this time. I would lie in the dark and listen to Josh along the corridor, moving a glass on his bedside cabinet, switching a lamp on and off, crying. The blue light from his phone would peep from the crack in the door and I knew that even if I could sleep, I would not. I felt guilty that my brain might allow for sleep when it was all my son craved. It would have been like eating in front of a starving man, unthinkable.

Here's the thing, I didn't know how to acknowledge the monster; it held me hostage. I didn't know what to say to it. Whether to stand tall and confront him like the unwanted intruder he was – that terrible thing that had got his hooks into my son. I avoided using the word depression, but kept to general terms, 'Josh is poorly' and 'it's not a good day . . .', thinking that if I didn't invite the word into our home it might not take root.

I didn't know how to tackle the monster, none of us did. This occurred to me daily, the thought that I should retaliate, grab my boy and roar, but this sparked fear that the monster might have got madder or roared louder than me, pushing Josh to do the unthinkable and taking him from me forever. And then how would I have coped? I was already bowed and fragile from living with the beast for too long when everything I used to consider routine was now disturbed or destroyed. To continue to ignore the monster felt easiest, but did little for my self-esteem and my shattered confidence, the fading belief that I could, with Simeon by my side, always do what was right for our little family, do what I needed to do to keep them safe.

I kept secrets from the monster too. I didn't tell him how I was more afraid of him than anyone or anything I had ever encountered in my whole life. Why? Because his arms were wrapped around the person I loved the most. He had Josh in his grip and there he sat, whispering in my son's ear and stoking the fire of his insecurities. I became a cowering shadow of the former me. Because what was at stake was my son. I kept a smiling face and swallowed the nausea that threatened. My hands shook and my head pounded. I was tired. I was beaten. I was low. I used to cry in the bath every night and I'd cry in the shower every morning. I hated that the person I loved did the monster's bidding.

It felt like a tug of war between me and him – the prize being Josh.

I fantasised about screaming at it, yelling at Josh:

'GET OUT OF MY HOUSE, GET YOUR HANDS OFF HIM!'

But I dared not – as I honestly couldn't have predicted who would win – and yet . . . until the moment I realised the monster had crept over our threshold and taken up residence, discreetly, silently, I truly believed that when it came to my boy, I could conquer any foe!

I kept other secrets.

I didn't confess that if the phone didn't get answered, my heart skipped and my imagination conjured such terrible images that they can make me weep even now – I pictured scenarios that are simply too frightening to voice, but ones where Josh was lost, taken, succumbed . . . and I was broken.

And I sob even now as I write these lines, having to admit that mixed with the drum of fear that beat in my heart was the creeping thought that if the worst *did* happen, at least the one I loved would be suffering no more. And maybe that was for the best. God, what a thought. What a terrible, terrible thought! That this might have been his very best option! At its worst his suffering made mine pale into insignificance, of course, and that is a reminder I find useful. For him it was and is a relentless battle.

The only thing I knew for certain is that I will never, ever give up on him.

Never.

This is a hard thing to admit, but I have wished that his suffering were physical. I of course wish he had *no* suffering at all, but if he has to suffer I thought this might be preferable.

Can you imagine a scenario where you would wish for your child any disease? No. Neither could I until depression came to live in our house, as insidious as any illness that attacks bones and tissue, but sneakier, harder to pin down and seemingly without the guaranteed cure we all so desperately crave. And the thing that's hardest of all is that the person you are trying to cure is only going through the motions, as if not fussed about a cure at all, almost as if he is on the opposing team!

Not consciously, but because he is lost to this illness.

It makes me want to weep and it makes me want to scream and beat the walls with my fists.

'Come on, Josh! Come on! We can't do this on our own! You need to help us, you need to help me!'

Yes, depression came to live in our house. It covered the windows in a dark shadow that gave the place a permanent air of night and sucked the joy from all the rooms so that Simeon and I, sleep-deprived, bickered in the half-light and Ben preferred to be anywhere but home.

It pulled down the blinds and blocked out the light.

It blocked out all of the light.

Chapter Eighteen

Josh

'So here it is, Merry Christmas!'

'I have been bent and broken, but – I hope – into a better shape.'

Charles Dickens

I had been taking Mirtazapine for a few weeks and with each day that passed I hoped I was going to start feeling the positive effects. Something, anything to justify the bloated, sleeping thing that I had become. I was, however, so foggy it was hard for me to tell if they were doing their job. The disappointment of each day without an upturn was like a scythe to any suggestion of optimism.

I had been home for about six weeks when the weather turned cold and I was vaguely aware of Christmas approaching but without any stirring of excitement or anticipation. If anything I just wanted it to be over. This was yet another marker for how far I had fallen from what was considered 'normal'. I haven't always dreaded the festive period. Only a few Christmases prior I was on the viewing platform of the Empire State Building on Christmas Eve when it started snowing and I have to admit that even I felt the 'magic' of the holiday season. That feeling was only a hazy memory now, like looking back on your own experiences through a shattered mirror, misted up by the steam of depression.

Being in the midst of severe depression and taking drugs that did very little to positively aid my illness felt like living in a time warp. When I look back I can't distinguish one day from another.

Every day was sad.

Every day was the same.

Every day was exhausting.

I pretty much stopped talking. Not only did I feel like I had nothing to say, but I didn't want to hear anyone else's thoughts either – my own were hard enough to deal with and I thought my silence would invite less comment. Mum and Simeon kept asking if I would go back to see the psychiatrist. I could see they were keen to return to something, possibly the only thing, that had been positive or at least had an effect on me. I didn't want to go back, unable to see how talking to him or anyone might help me. I felt like an observer as the rest of the family came and went and chatted across the table and it was often a surprise when they addressed me directly, because I often felt as if I was invisible, and this reminded me that I could be seen.

I had minimal contact with the outside world other than watching YouTube videos, watching Twitch streams and listening to podcasts on Audible.

My friends were understandably ill-equipped to cope with my illness. I didn't address them directly, but as Ben and I shared a similar friendship group, I know they would have been aware. I don't hold this against them, not at all – *I* was too ill-equipped to handle it, not that I had much choice. I was too fucked-up to envy them the fact that they were busy with the job of being in their twenties and all that went with that. Normal life was so remote from how I existed; it took the biggest effort to wake up and on most days I couldn't make it to the shower. This state of affairs went from being something I chose to something that I was anxious about to the point where going outside the house, let alone interacting with people, filled me with dread.

It was like living in a fog that made my actions sluggish and my thoughts erratic. Looking back, I can see that this was probably the scariest time for me. I was stuck at home where my whole world was a fourteen-by-sixteen-foot box. I knew I had depression. I knew I was ill, but what I didn't know and what no one could tell me was if or when my sharp thoughts were going to return. The ability to think in the way I did had always been my one good thing. My body might have let me down often, but my brain . . . I couldn't conceive of a life without clarity of thought and the constant jump of ideas that had been my norm. If I felt the beginnings of anything at all it was anger and impatience; both of these I can now see were a positive step that slowly began edging out the numbness. But of course I didn't recognise that at the time.

The atmosphere in the house was strained to say the least. Sleeping, for me, was no longer about sleep, it was about escape and it was a state of exhaustion that no amount of sleep could fix. Being in bed with my eyes closed was the only way I knew how to survive. When the battle is to stay awake or keep your eyes open or even look at another human, being told to go for a 'nice' walk or 'meet up with friends' is the equivalent of someone suggesting you climb Mount Everest and do star jumps on the summit for weight loss. I wished people would stop making suggestions – they clearly had no clue as to what I was going through. Nearly everyone who came to the house, friends and family, suggested in so many variants:

'Why don't you go for a little walk?'
'Shall we go on a walk?'
'Fancy a walk, Joshy?'

'How about a stroll, a bit of fresh air?'

And each time I had to politely refuse made me feel like shit. Not only did I not have the energy for a walk, but the fact that they just didn't get it only added to my sense of isolation.

I stuck with the Mirtazapine, thinking that my body would get used to it, desperate for the change I'd imagined. I knew that the psychiatrist had confirmed that there were as many variables in drugs and dosages as there were people with depression, but I believed, illogically, that things would plateau. With hindsight, I can see that was not going to happen but I was locked in a spiral – the drugs were the only thing on offer and so I took them. It felt better to be doing *something* and once I had started taking them, I didn't want to believe they weren't working and that I had gone through the horror of their side effects for nothing, so I kept taking them . . .

Christmas came and went. It was awful. The house was full of people, noisy people, and all I wanted was silence. I've never been a huge fan of Christmas hits, but at that point the sound of jingling bells and jolly lyrics were like a hammer on an anvil inside my skull. I remember leaving my bed to venture downstairs and feeling overwhelmed by the number of people in the house, many of them rushing at me with gifts.

It was all too much, all too much.

I walked into the sitting room and it seemed packed with people, all with drinks and wearing Christmas jumpers or sparkly clothes, the atmosphere was one of fun and celebration. I felt as if they all looked up, alerted by my presence, and the atmosphere changed, becoming quiet and solemn, as if the elephant had come downstairs and was now quite literally in the room.

I didn't join them for Christmas lunch, but could hear their con-versation floating up through the floorboards and into my room. I had a sandwich in my room and cried and slept. I remember sloping back up the stairs in my pyjamas and could see one or two people scowling as if I was being rude but that was just too fucking bad. I couldn't help but think that had things gone my way only a month or so before I would not have even been there for Christmas – this no more than a cursory thought. I like this reminder taken from 'Depression and Christmas' advice from The Priory: 'Society drums into us the idea that Christmas is a time of joy, laughter, cheerfulness and partying. However, for people who struggle with depression, the constant reminder that you should be happy can make you feel even worse.'[13]

In the New Year, Mum and Simeon went to clear out and hand over the studio in Southampton and I knew I had to tell them about what I believed was stashed under the mattress.

I called Simeon into my room – I was nervous, but I knew the discovery would be more than Mum could handle – and said, 'When you go into my flat, there is something I need you to get from under my mattress.' I then tried to find the words to explain that I had bought suicide pills. It was hard. My tongue stuck to the roof of my mouth.

Simeon shook his head. 'You don't have to tell me, Joshy.'

'I do,' I pressed. 'I do because—'

'No, son. I know what you are talking about and I found them that day I came to bring you home. I brought them back here and flushed them down the loo.'

'Does Mum know?'

Simeon nodded.

It felt weird to know that they had had the full picture all along, relieving in some ways. I was also aware that they could have reacted so differently, got angry or gone nuts, interrogated me, but they did none of these things and I felt glad that they had been calm. It was at moments like these that I realised how lucky I was to have them as my parents; they might not have always 'got it' and Mum certainly drove me to distraction, but they never stopped trying to understand and do the right thing.

Chapter Nineteen

Amanda

'Peter Peter Poinsettia!'

'When you love someone, you love the person as they are, and not as you'd like them to be.'

Leo Tolstoy

There was only a matter of weeks between Josh arriving home from university after the worst episode when Simeon discovered the pills and the arrival of Christmas. I had the entire family coming to our house. I wanted it to be perfect and was again running blind, feeling my way and was so completely out of control that I didn't know what to do. I went to Asda to do a big food shop and remember standing at the end of the checkout with bags opened, but with so much running through my mind, I forgot to pack my groceries. Items were piling up around the bags, and I just stared. It was chaotic and I couldn't figure out what to do. I was tired, distracted and tearful. A woman in the queue behind me barged forward and started shoving the things I had bought into the bags – 'Here you go, hun!' she sneered at me – and I watched as mince pies were squashed under litres of milk and fruit was lobbed in on top. Her sarcasm and passive aggression was more than I could handle. I picked up my handbag and walked away. Leaving her shouting at the poor cashier who didn't really know what to do next.

At this time, arguably when Josh needed comfort most, if I reached out for him he would physically swerve as though my very touch was toxic, as if I might only make things worse and that any contact might break the splendid state of isolation in which he existed. I became a bit nervous about seeing him as he would scowl at me or stare at me blankly and I didn't know how to respond. I felt useless. Simeon could only tell me that things would settle down and Ben avoided coming home. Some bloody Christmas!

I hoped that by the time Christmas Day arrived, the anti-depressants might have started to have a positive effect and also thought that the diversion of Christmas might be good for Josh.

It wasn't.

And I know now that this was a misfire on my part. I guess it was also a way for me to escape the sour bubble in which we were entombed – when you live in a small space it is hard to escape the suffocating nature of depression, even if it is not you who is depressed. And if I think about it, I suppose I was trying to be a good mum for Ben and a good wife to Simeon as well as trying to make up for the fact that I had not been there when I was needed.

I decided to make the house look as festive as possible. I stocked the fridge with goodies and took care to wrap the usual socks, pants and aftershave prettily. My plan was that I might then be able to distract everyone from the monster who had by now firmly taken up residence in our home. My Christmas preparation was the equivalent of the photographer clicking his fingers with the right hand while snapping away with his left.

I was smiling and desperate to make the holiday season the best it could be for our other son, our parents, the wider family and the young nieces and nephews, who of course deserved to feel the magic. It wasn't their fault we had the dark, unwanted monster in residence. All the little ones cared about was eating sweets and playing charades. It wasn't Josh's fault either and yet he was the one who spent much of the festivities cloistered away in his bedroom, as if exiled, seeking solace on the mattress that had become his firm-sprung island refuge.

He would appear from time to time, his tall frame awkwardly filling the doorway, as if uncertain how to greet people, where to sit and possibly aware for the first time that, unlike every other guest dolled up in their Sunday best, he was in his pyjamas or his underwear. His hair was unwashed, his breath tainted, skin sallow and his eyes vacant.

It tore at my heart.

The family would rush to greet him:

'It's Joshy!'

'Hello, Josh!'

'Happy Christmas, darling!'

'We've missed you!'

'Love you, Joshy!'

'Come and sit here!'

'What can we get you to eat?'

Prior to their arrival, we had told our immediate family of the situation, watching as each of their faces fell in distress, immediately followed by the question 'What can we do to help him?' And if their sincere words and affirmations of love were able to heal, he would have cartwheeled down the hallway and burst into song. But I knew for a fact that even had the words been bullets, he was armoured, resilient, and nothing could puncture the shell depression had coated our boy with. Their words slid from his sadness and pooled on the floor for us to slip in.

Josh would stare at the people who looked at him with such expressions of expectation. He seemed overwhelmed and anxious. Once or twice he waved at the kids, might even have kissed his grandparents, but more often than not he would grab a glass of water from the kitchen and slope back up the stairs.

At the sound of his bedroom door firmly closing, my mum would cry. My dad would sit with misty eyes, Simeon and I would exchange a look of utter, utter helplessness, and Ben would creep back to his room. And still the questions raced around and around endlessly like a motorcyclist in the wall of death – *How can we make him better? What are we supposed to be doing? How long can we all live like this?*

Whilst trying to turn the house into a festive wonderland, I bought a poinsettia, not my favourite plant by any stretch of the imagination and post-Christmas I positively detest them. I mention this darned plant because in the midst of trying to cope with my son's mental illness I did some pretty crazy things. These included: praying to a God I do not believe exists. Buying statues and pictures of other deities I also do not believe exist and to which I prayed on a daily basis, asking them all to help me figure out how to make Josh better. Giving large sums to charity in the hope that karma is a real thing. Oh, and anthropomorphising that bloody poinsettia.

Yes, you read that correctly.

I didn't say it was logical.

Or made sense.

I mention it only because I think it perfectly demonstrates the desperate helplessness I felt, based on the very real fear that if and when my son decided to end his life there was absolutely nothing I could do about it. This fear that punched me in the gut several times a day meant I had to learn how to act, smiling and laughing on TV or the radio, while my stomach twisted at the simple fact that I was useless when it came to protecting and defending the person I loved most.

I put the poinsettia – for argument's sake let's call him . . . Peter. (Okay, I actually *did* call him Peter, but put this fact in as if a witty afterthought because I didn't want you to think I was losing my grip on reality – see how this stigma/shame thing works?) Peter was purchased to add a warm splash of red colour to an otherwise dull windowsill in the TV room – how could he not fail to lift Josh's spirits?

I walked into the room one day and Josh was asleep on the sofa where he had lain for a few days, as usual only leaving to pee, drink and eat toast. During this time, Simeon and I left him to it, not sitting down to watch TV because we didn't want to wake Josh. It was one example of how his illness took something from us, the small ability to sit on the couch with a cup of tea and watch a telly programme. It was one of a thousand tiny disruptions to family life that led to a low-level feeling of resentment. And believe it or not, seeing him asleep on the sofa was a small moment of celebration because when your child's world is reduced to a bed, the fact that he had made it to the sofa was a good, good thing.

Peter was, I noticed, looking decidedly droopy, and this with a week or so to go until Christmas Day. I watered him and might have offered some gentle words of encouragement.

'Come on, Peter, don't give up. You are pretty and bright and will make Christmas wonderful.'

Having gone about my chores I stripped the beds and cleaned the bathroom before popping my head in on Josh and . . . miracle upon miracles, he was sitting up! And not only sitting up, he seemed quite awake and mentally present. To see this small lift in his demeanour, to find him alert, made my spirit soar. I was, as ever when these moments occurred, keen to harness the moment and see if I could glean a little insight into his state of mind that might help me when he again slipped back to sleep or, worse, appeared in the doorway in his pants with that vacant stare.

I knelt down on the rug and smiled at him.

'Hey, Josh. How are you doing right now?'

'Imokay.' His standard response.

'Can I get you anything that might make you more comfortable?'

He shook his head and pulled the blanket up under his chin.

'Well, I'll check on you again in a bit, and if you want anything at all, or you just want to chat. Shout out.'

'Imokay.'

It was as I stood to leave that I saw Peter Poinsettia on the windowsill and he was positively perky. His leaves arched proudly towards the light and the deep red colour seemed more vibrant than ever. New shoots stood proud from the stem and Josh followed my line of sight.

'Plant looks good.' He spoke in gravelled tones from a voice ill used to being exercised.

I nodded and was overtaken by a thought that was, as I said earlier, most illogical. And it was this: if I could keep Peter healthy, if Peter did not die, then neither would Josh. It was as if this garish plant in its gaudy gold pot was in some way a barometer for all that was going on with Josh.

I dashed downstairs, flipped open my laptop and just as I had done when searching for guidance on how to care for a depressed child, I read all I could about how to keep poinsettias healthy. I learned about the right amount of water, the soil depth, how much sunlight/shade was best and I resolved to keep Peter in tip-top condition.

And I did.

For months and months and months . . .

There was one near miss when I was working in a London studio to record one of my audiobooks and was away from the house

196

for six days straight. I came home and dashed straight up the stairs to find Josh was asleep. I was distressed to see that Peter was flagging. I burst into tears and cradled him to me, taking him to the kitchen sink where I tenderly removed the small browning, crispy leaves and watched in dismay as some healthier looking leaves simply dropped off at my touch. I gave him water and told him that even though Christmas had come and gone, he was still valued and added beauty to an otherwise dull room.

'Why are you crying?' Simeon asked from the hallway.

'My plant nearly died!' I explained.

'It's only a plant.' He stared at me nonplussed. 'Are you tired, love? Why don't you go to sleep?'

'Imokay.' I borrowed the catchall and it seemed to do the trick. I managed to stop myself from screaming out loud:

IT'S NOT JUST A PLANT! IT'S PETER! AND I HAVE TO KEEP HIM ALIVE BECAUSE ON THE DAY HE PERKED UP, JOSH WOKE UP AND SAT UP AND I CAN'T EXPLAIN WHY BUT I THINK THEY ARE CONNECTED AND I CAN'T LET ETIHER OF THEM WILT OR FLAG OR SHRIVEL UP – IT'S UP TO ME. I HAVE TO KEEP THEM ALIVE!

You can see how '*Imokay*' felt easier.

As time went on, I asked Josh to help me take care of Peter and he did, on occasion, water him and tend to him and it brought me such joy! I know I slept easier on those nights.

It was during this time that Simeon would hold me tight each and every night as I cried myself to sleep and he would then take my hand in his where our arms formed a V across the mattress: so I knew he was there, just in case. I would sleep for a few hours before waking with a jolt in the wee small hours, as if suddenly remembering I had left the iron on or forgotten to close a window. It was with that same heart-thumping sense that all was not right with the world that I would throw off the duvet and creep from the room, making my way across the landing to Josh's room. I would find him either asleep, coiled as if in pain, or awake, with the light of his device lighting up his face in the darkness as he watched endless YouTube videos or binge-watched box sets; anything, anything to pass the endless tedium of night. He would barely react to my presence, so much so that I would have to peer really closely to see if he was awake or asleep. Ironically, he told me that he wished for night to pass so he could greet the dawn and stay in bed all day to sleep/doze/watch mindless YouTube videos and box sets so as to quickly reach night-time . . . you get the message. It was for him an endless cycle of trying to make time pass or trying to make time stop.

One night, he looked up at me as I stood in the doorway and said, 'I can't do this anymore, Mum.'

My heart raced. I thought he was telling me that he wanted to give up, check out, and I felt the rise of panic as I struggled to form the sentence that might be the balm to his hurt. His next words, however, were like a symphony to my ears.

'I can't keep taking this medication and feeling like this. I want to come off the tablets.'

'Yes, Joshy! Whatever you think is best. We need to find out how to do that and what happens next, but, yes, whatever you think . . .'

I practically skipped back to bed and woke Simeon. Not only had Josh engaged with me, but he was talking about taking action, making a change that showed he had his future in mind. This was HUGE and the very first time in over a year that he had shown any willingness to rely on his own thoughts or decision-making. I settled back on the pillows and when I looked at the monster sitting at the foot of our bed, he looked a little smaller and a little afraid.

'That's right, you fucker! I am going to win!'

'What did you say?' Simeon asked in a sleepy haze.

'Nothing, darling. Night-night.'

Chapter Twenty

Josh

'And another fresh start . . .'

'Fall if you will, but rise you must.'

James Joyce

It came upon me very suddenly: the thought that I did not want to continue on medication, any medication. I didn't want to carry on living like this. My existence was pointless, based on being asleep more than I was awake. And when I was awake I felt so foggy it was like I wasn't present. It was no life. I couldn't remember the most basic things I was asked or told. My brain was mush. Pointless. I was a zombie, otherworldly, out of whack, and I knew deep down that if I carried on like that I was going to get lost, possibly forever, and that thought terrified me more than any other.

Looking back, this realisation was a massive step in the right direction. Regardless of whether medication was the right or wrong path for me to take, it was the first step towards regaining control. I looked at the pill in my hand and the blister pack in the other containing next month's dosage and I literally had to force myself to put the tablet in my mouth and swallow. It was like there was a small voice inside me, the voice of reason that had been lost for quite some time, and it was making me question: *Why are you taking these, Josh? Do you think they are helping?* And the answer was that I didn't know why I was still taking them and no, they weren't helping.

I suspected they were doing me more harm than good and knew that if they were going to make a positive difference they probably would have by now. I had hoped that the medication would work by giving me a short-term break that would alleviate the worst aspects of my depression. I wanted them to do what they did for others: take the edge off my extreme sadness and mute my suicidal feelings. The problem for me was that they also muted everything else, to the point where I was a walking shell. If Citalopram was for me a sticking plaster then Mirtazapine was a suture, and the trouble was that the wound underneath was no closer to healing and that was my problem. Tablets weren't the cure I was looking for. They were a mask: a useful mask undoubtedly, and I can see that for those who manage to get the drug and dosage right, it might be a way to live with depression, but not for me.

In recent months I have looked at the use of antidepressants and understand that for millions and millions of people they *are* the thing that brings them back from the brink, takes the edge off their depression and allows them to function. I have spoken to a lot of sufferers who work, play sport and enjoy a family life on medication, 'functioning depressives' if you like, and they are convinced it's all down to the medication that helps alter their brain chemistry.

When you are suffering from depression, finding the right combination of drug and dose can feel a bit hit and miss and this at a time when what you need most is change, quick change, but there is nothing quick about getting better from depression, it is like turning a tanker, slow and steady, and often you don't realise it's turning until the operation is well underway. According to the *Guardian*, in the UK 'More than 7.3 million people were prescribed antidepressants in 2017–18, 4.4 million of whom also received a prescription for such drugs in both of the two previous years.' And '1.6 million people prescribed antidepressants in the past year were "new" users', meaning they were not prescribed such drugs in previous years.[14]

In the USA, *Time* magazine reported – citing a report from the National Center for Health Statistics – that 'Close to 13 per cent of people twelve and older said they took an antidepressant in the last month. That number is up from 11 per cent in 2005–2008 . . . a 65 per cent increase since 1999–2002, when 7.7 per cent of Americans reported taking an antidepressant.'[15]

It feels important to say that everyone's depression journey is different and there is no one-size-fits-all treatment or solution. Sadly, there is only what works for you, and if medication is the treatment that makes life possible then I can only envy you that.

I became aware that I had very little recollection of the past few months. This moment of clarity, as I stood at the sink with the pill on my tongue, rose up like a bright thing in the gloom and was in itself a breakthrough. I thought back to a time when my isolation was self-imposed, but in the last few months, since taking the drugs, I had been overwhelmed by a debilitating fatigue that dogged me morning, noon and night. I knew with these muddied thoughts it would be impossible to get a mental foothold that would allow me to get back to normal, or if not back to normal, then at least help me improve. Somewhere in the back of my mind I knew that I had little hope of recovery while I was in this state.

I had mentioned it to Mum the night before, but this time I told her, 'I don't want to take these anymore. They are killing me.'

She was supportive but concerned and pointed out that I could not just stop, it was *bad* for me to just stop.

I actually laughed out loud.

'Bad for me? What, worse than wanting to jump off a bridge or take a handful of pills? Worse than feeling like I'm not on the planet? Worse than sleeping my entire life away?'

For fuck's sake, there was so much about my life at that point that was '*bad for me*' it was hard to know where the good lay.

On my psychiatrist's advice I halved the dose I had been taking and he suggested I do this for a week. Mum and Simeon were really worried and Mum insisted she kept me with her, so when she went to London for a long-standing arrangement to stay with my aunt and uncle, I grudgingly went too. It took all of my courage to shower and leave the house. It felt so strange being outside, surreal. The air was cold on my face, the sky too bright. The world felt alien to me and very loud. I tried to block out the noise and suppress my nausea by putting my earphones on and closing my eyes and I spent the whole train journey like that. We arrived at Paddington Station and my desire to be sick overwhelmed me. The moment I stepped from the train I ran outside to find a bin, my skin felt clammy. I was in a cold sweat and was so sick I threw up my stomach lining. I could hardly stand up – I was dizzy and faint and wished I were back at home in bed. Mum was near to tears and we jumped in a cab with all the windows down and her repeating, 'Nearly there, Joshy, nearly there . . .' while the taxi driver asked repeatedly, 'He's not going to be sick, is he?', and Mum reassuring him, 'No he won't, and anyway I have a bag ready.'

Funny that even though my head swam and my limbs were shaking, I can recall his annoyance, his tuts.

I fell into bed at my Uncle Paul and Auntie Stevie's flat and slept the day and night away. I knew they were pleased to see me and wanted to interact, catch up, chat, but this was beyond me. I was too preoccupied with fielding the effects of withdrawal. And it was far from pleasant. I don't know what I had expected, but in the way that the drugs had had a gradual effect on my mental and physical health when I began taking them, I guessed withdrawing from them might be similar. It was not. My physical reaction was brutal and almost unbearable. I craved Mirtazapine, actually missing the taste of it, which sounds odd now as I write it. I lay on a sweat-soaked sheet and the room spun. I felt grubby and wished I were in my own bed next to my own shower. It felt like having motion sickness. I even took motion-sickness tablets, thinking they might make a difference. They didn't.

Mum reluctantly left early the next morning to go to work. I felt horrific: it was like I had the flu, but with the shakes, sickness and a headache that was blinding. The room continued to spin and I called her up and asked her to come back. She was near to tears, explaining that she had no transport and was at the mercy of those she was travelling with who, of course, did not fully understand the situation. She told me that someone reassured her by saying, 'Oh, he'll be okay, he's a big boy!'

But I didn't feel like a big boy. I felt like an adult in crisis and an adult who was slipping away. And I was scared.

I had to wait a couple of hours for her to return. I lay on the bed in the strange room and did not know what to do with myself. Again, I was in a cold sweat and was losing grip of which way was up.

It became clear my current low dose was not a good idea – who knew? When we got home that night, I took three quarters of a tablet and I continued this for the next week or so, then I lowered it to half a tablet and then a quarter and so on. I did this until the tablets ran out and I didn't get any more.

That was it.

I was drug-free.

It took a few weeks more for me to lose the effects of the drugs, until the foggy head and extreme fatigue and appetite spikes settled, and when they did . . . well, it won't come as a surprise to know that I felt exactly as I had before I started taking the drugs. What did I expect? I don't know. But I do know I was disappointed to be back to square one: depressed and frustrated. The question was, what was I going to do now?

Everyone in the family kept telling me how well I had done to quit my medication. I think they rightly saw it as the first step to me taking control, the first step towards getting the old Josh back, which was true. The downside was they also expected, based on nothing more than the amount of time that had passed, me to be getting 'better' and with this came a whole new wave of questioning:

'So, what now, Josh?'

'Do you want to go back to university?'

'Might you get a job?'

On and on it went, the endless suggestions and questions from my well-meaning family and friends, who seemed to feel my inactivity to be a great irritation, as if they too were disappointed and expected me to be a little ray of sunshine. I didn't know what to say to them, nothing polite anyway. Did they think I was fixed? Their lack of understanding of the condition was and is so bloody annoying.

On a positive note, I *had* managed to quit my medication, which felt like a small win and I hoped it might be a springboard to better mental health. Things obviously hadn't worked out for me in Southampton and I began to think that maybe a fresh start in a new place away from the hellish memories of my lowest point might be the thing I needed to get back on track.

I thought that it might have been the place, the isolation of Southampton, that had contributed to my depression and figured that if I stayed close to home, I might be able to get my degree after all. I could not envisage a future that did not involve the world of science and knew that a degree was the only way to gain entry.

It was on a good day, a month or so later, one where I was able to get out of bed, shower, eat breakfast and chat to Mum and Simeon that I applied to Bristol University to read Biological Sciences, and knowing my history they offered me a place on the proviso that I went into the halls of residence so that a senior resident was on hand. It felt like a vote of confidence and yet again I imagined completing my studies and leaving with the piece of paper that would be the ticket to a bright future. I started to think that everything might just click into place. I hoped so.

I had to fill out the standard University and Colleges Admission Service form and remember being paralysed with fear, unable to type or enter my details, sick with anxiety and aware that if I didn't fill out the form, I would not be able to take a place. Looking back, I think this was a sign that I was far from ready, far from 'well enough', and yet I chose to ignore this warning. I filled out the form, eventually.

Mum and Simeon kept telling me that this was my chance to start over, a new environment, a new course, and yet still close enough to the safety net of home should I fall down again. I had heard this before. It sounds perfect, doesn't it? And it might have been, were it not for that damned depression that still lurked in every corner of my mind. To remind them of this felt negative, like I was giving up or not being a glass-half-full kinda guy. I could see they so wanted me to be better, beaming when I managed to hold a conversation with my grandparents, smiling at each other when I joined them at the dinner table and almost apoplectic with joy if I said I was going to see my friends. Their relief was tangible.

So I kept quiet, my favourite head-in-the-sand action, and tried to figure out how to go forward.

I was still sick and any brightening in my demeanour, any sense of hope I gave out, was in fact only a hiatus. It was, I can see now, only a matter of time until my illness peaked again, because the reality was I was playing at being 'better'. In the early hours, in my favourite 3 a.m. world, I was still driven by thoughts of how to end my life. I tried to quiet them, but it was hard. It was an exhausting rollercoaster, a rollercoaster with a ticking time bomb under my seat.

My parents decided that to celebrate this new chapter and the general uplift in everyone's mood, we should take a family holiday before the start of the new term and so in the August of 2017 they booked a trip to Florida to put us all on an actual rollercoaster – to say I had my reservations would be an understatement.

That whole trip was like a living nightmare. In fact, if you tried to conjure my perfect nightmare it would consist of unbearable heat, dense crowds, constant screaming and being forced to live shoulder to shoulder with my family and their friends under one roof while we all tried to have the very best time! I was on edge and know this was infectious for the rest of the group, which then made my anxiety and guilt rear their ugly heads, which meant I was in a low mood and this put me more on edge. It was like being on the shittiest emotional merry-go-round imaginable.

Each day the house woke with squeals of excitement about what was happening, where we would visit and what the plans were, and each day I would have to steel myself to get out of bed and go and join in the party. There were moments of happiness – seeing my little cousin's face beam when he met the 'real' Transformers and a couple of laughs at Universal Studios – but I knew that if it took that much effort for me to feel happy in a large, sunny theme park in Florida – a situation many would consider to be the best and happiest place ever – well, that only made me worried for what might be around the corner when I returned to the world of higher education in a less sunny place. And that came round quick enough.

We had been back from Florida for a month or so when I felt a strong sense of déjà vu as I entered another hall of residence. My irritation levels rose as Mum strung up fairy lights and put plants on the shelves. I did, however, see the happiness in her eyes when only a few days later I told her I had been out with new friends and had even attended a lecture. I think I knew deep down that it was only a matter of time before the smile was once again wiped from her face and we would be back to square one. But I kept quiet, of course I did. I so wanted it to work out, for me, for my parents, my grandparents, for everyone who had seen me sink so low. We didn't really talk directly about what had happened in Southampton – it felt like the hardest of conversations to have and, I'm sure, to be reminded of it felt like opening an old wound, but it was a wound that was not yet healed for me and painful because of it.

Bristol University had a system in place whereby a senior resident lived among new students, effectively providing a door to knock on if a crisis should arise. The senior resident in the block was a student himself, only a year or so older than me, and in all honesty, even though he was a really nice bloke, he was not, in my opinion, trained well enough to handle any real emergency. He was a bit quiet, shy even, and was either engrossed in his studies or not there. I don't think this system was quite the mental health safety net the university felt it was. There was also a warden on site who was a little out of touch and fixated on things that I felt were of no importance, while the really serious stuff seemed to go over his head.

I can't write this book without referencing the high suicide rate at Bristol University. I can't and won't attempt to explain the reasons behind it, which are many and complex, but I do know the university and those responsible for pastoral care are taking notice.

The students themselves are galvanised and I sincerely hope this greater awareness, along with cooperation in The University Mental Health Charter will mean different outcomes for future students.

Students, aware of the high numbers of suicides, are starting to demand more support. Organisers of a protest by Bristol University students said there was a 'growing mental health crisis' at the university. And according to a BBC news report, 'In Bristol the number of students seeking help has risen by 106 per cent in the past five years – from 1,375 in 2012–13 to 2,827 in 2016–17.'[16]

I was glad to have the support of family close by. I also met a great group of people who I liked hanging out with, the kind of friends you have for life and who are still the people I turn to. My friends were aware of my mental health battle. I felt awkward telling them, still the words tasted of shame, but I plucked up the courage and did so one night after a couple of beers. Thankfully they took my revelation in their stride and I am glad I told them. It has meant that they are aware of my need to sometimes disappear and gather my thoughts or my preference to be alone, and they look out for me in the way I do them.

Despite having this new level of support, the demons of anxiety and low self-esteem started to whisper in my ear and it wasn't long before I started to self-medicate with alcohol. Being drunk was a welcome release. And while living in the halls of residence, it was still my go-to activity when it came to taking a break from the intensity of my condition. I can now see that this was almost a repetition of my behaviour in Southampton, but I was too scared to think about that.

The simple truth was, I might have been able to leave my bed each day and I had certainly repackaged myself, grown my hair, changed university, but my brain didn't care about those things. I was still slowly falling apart, wary of messing up this second and possibly last chance that I had been given to study and yet without the ability to concentrate or focus. My life was erratic and only mirrored what was going on inside my head. I was either drinking or sleeping.

Mum and Simeon, indeed the whole family, were so chuffed that I had a place at Bristol that to tell them I felt like I was sinking was not an option. I wanted this to be my shot as much as they did. I wanted nothing more than to put the last few years behind me and get back to 'normal', whatever that means. Not that they were overtly pressuring me, but it was their subtle hints offered unconsciously, about '*how proud*' they were and '*how great it was*' to see me getting back on my feet and '*I knew you could do it, Josh!*' that left me in no doubt that to hear I wanted to leave, again, would be a blow to them all.

As the first semester progressed, I began to drink heavily. Very heavily. It wasn't unusual for me to drink a small bottle of vodka before going out and then consume ten pints of cider or beer until I passed out. I sought the oblivion that being drunk offered. I liked it. I liked it very much. The escape alcohol offered was very attractive. I knew I was heading for a fall and I did not give a shit.

Chapter Twenty-One

Amanda

'The crossroads'

'One swallow does not make a summer, neither does one fine day; similarly one day or brief time of happiness does not make a person entirely happy.'

Aristotle

The months idled by and with Josh settled into his first year at Bristol University, and Ben now studying up in Liverpool, we found the forever house which we had been dreaming of since I first put pen to paper in 2011 and wrote my first novel *Poppy Day*. When I wrote the story of a young girl whose husband is taken hostage in Afghanistan and her incredible efforts to bring home the man she loves, figuring no one would fight for his freedom like she does, we were living in a grotty army quarter with a leaky roof and army standard-issue furniture. We daydreamed about how if ever my writing career took off we would buy a rambling, rundown farmhouse with creaky floors, wonky doors, real fires, an Aga and old flagstone floors in the kitchen. Many a rainy day was filled with how we would wander the garden in our pyjamas and wellington boots and watch the sunset with a cup of tea in our mitts, sitting on a tartan blanket. This had been our fantasy for a long time and the thought alone had warmed us on many a rainy day.

Suddenly, with money in the bank, the details of this house fell into our hands and it was love at first sight. We tentatively asked Josh what he thought about moving away, aware of how change could for him be unsettling and he told us quite openly that every time he walked into the house we lived in, he saw his depression and he felt it. And this made sense; it was after all the place where he had been the unhappiest. He was keen to go to a new house and start over and not have to sleep in the bedroom that had been like a prison.

I had not fully considered this but it made absolute sense; it must have been like returning to the scene of an accident every single day. That was it, decision made. Our offer was accepted and we waited for the usual legal shenanigans to take place so we could move in and make it our dream home. I was beyond excited.

We began packing up our little house in preparation for our move out to the countryside. Josh had, by this stage, taken the massive first steps on the road to recovery and was awake more than he was asleep. I even threw Peter Poinsettia away before the move! Just binned him – and it felt great. We were incredibly proud of how Josh had started back at university and one a lot, lot closer to home. It meant we could be by his side within half an hour if he should feel himself slipping, and yet it gave him an outlet, a purpose, the chance to focus on something other than his depression. We figured that if he could get back to studying, who knew where that might lead? We were so very proud of his strength, determination and independence. Not that he was out of the woods, not by a long shot, but if the monster had had Josh firmly in his grip, it was now

211

relegated to sitting in the corner, giving Josh the freedom to look up for the first time in an age.

Moving into halls seemed like a good way to reacquaint himself with life outside the house and also to get him back into student life in a slightly more monitored way. He quickly made a group of wonderful friends, which was something that thrilled me, and he of course kept a couple of his old ones, but it was this new group, who saw Josh with fresh eyes that allowed him to shake off his old skin. He bought new clothes and took an interest in his appearance for the first time in as long as Simeon and I could remember.

Things were going . . . okay. Not great, but okay. Josh was much improved but was still a little withdrawn and introspective. Simeon and I had concerns about how Josh was living his life; yes, it was great he had a friendship group and, yes, wonderful that he had gone back to studying, but the heavy drinking and then coming home to sleep for days on end? It was a red flag to put it mildly and not how I wanted our son to live. We justified his behaviour because it was so good to have him up, dressed and living as part of the human race. It was all too easy to think back to the worst days when we would have given absolutely anything to have him out and about, but his lifestyle felt destructive and we were both now experienced enough to understand that it was a way of him dealing or rather *not* dealing with what was going on in his head.

Again he refused to speak to a professional and we were back to that horrible feeling that we were in limbo, fearful for our child but dealing with an adult. Simeon and I argued. We bickered over how to handle the situation. He was anxious that Josh was falling into bad old habits and was not addressing his mental state and predicted that he would in all likelihood crash again and leave without completing his studies. I disagreed and pointed out all the positives: Josh's new friendship group, the fact that we were on hand should he start to slide and how Josh seemed so happy to have his place at Bristol. It was a tense time for us as we were on different pages. I didn't like it one bit.

We decided to do what we had always done: keep the door for communication open, keep checking in on Josh and making sure he was as safe as possible. I thought about what Simeon had said and asked Josh about his studies. He was vague to say the least, and I got the distinct feeling not much academic work was going on. I wondered if Simeon was right, questioning for the first time whether maybe university simply wasn't for Josh, that maybe he was still not 'fixed' enough to slide back into everyday life and simply crack on! Had we made a mistake? I couldn't decide whether we had enabled his dream or pushed him into a nightmare. The sleepless nights returned for me, this time my thoughts were occupied with that age-old question: was Josh getting happier? And what were the conditions that might make him happy?

One night, I think it was in February after Josh had started in September, he called out of the blue, not to ask for a lift or to give us his rather précised update on how he was feeling, but to say that he didn't feel right. We were glad he felt able to make contact, but he was hesitant, quiet and it set every alarm bell ringing.

Without telling him, we jumped in the car and spoke to him as we drove to his halls of residence, wary of heightening the situation and making things awkward or embarrassing him in his halls or in front of his new friends, but at the same time wanting to be close to him, just in case . . . Simeon gave me knowing looks and in that moment we were on the exact same page: worried for our son.

'How are you feeling, Josh?' I asked, trying to make it sound almost casual, as Simeon drove the thirty minutes from our house to the halls of residence.

'I don't know.'

'Can you try and describe it, Joshy? Are you feeling good or bad?' I simplified it so as not to overtax a brain that might be struggling. My instinct told me he was in a bad place and it made my heart race. I pictured the tablets he had ordered before and I saw the headlines of another student who had succumbed to suicide, and another and another . . .

'Erm . . . not good,' he mumbled.

'So, bad. Okay, darling. Does it feel like you are struggling, Josh?' I asked, biting my lip and waiting for his response, which was slow in coming.

'Like I'm not coping. I'm very anxious,' he answered eventually.

'Okay, okay, well, just hang in there. Do you want to come home?'

'I don't think so. No. No I don't.'

'Well, we are coming to see you, just to talk. We are on our way.'

'No! I don't want you here. Don't come!' His tone immediately changed, he sounded furious and this frightened me as much as his slow, drawn-out responses. Simeon stared ahead, jaw clenched, trying to get there as quickly as he could.

'Okay, okay, keep as calm as you can. We won't come in, I promise' – I spoke slowly, calmly – 'but we *will* be sitting outside just in case. And we will stay outside in the car until either you feel a bit better or you think you might need to talk to someone or you fall asleep or you need us to bring you home or whatever. Just take your time. There's no rush, Josh, we have all the time in the world.'

'I don't want you here!'

'I hear you, Josh, but if you are in danger . . .'

'I'm not in danger!' He sounded adamant, but my gut told me he might be. I remembered what it had been like to take that call in Australia.

I had a tight ball of anxiety in my stomach and Simeon was driving with one ear cocked to the conversation, his knuckles white on the steering wheel.

'Do you think there's a chance you might kill yourself, Josh? Are you feeling suicidal right now?'

I had done it, said all the terrible words that had been cued up on my tongue since he called. It felt frightening to say it out loud and I was wary of putting the thought in his head. I didn't know if it was the wrong or right thing to do.

Silence.

'Josh, speak to me, love, do you think that tonight, you might try to kill yourself?' My voice was firm, commanding and yet on the inside my gut churned and my veins ran with pure liquid fear. Simeon reached over and squeezed my hand and it felt like the right thing to have done.

'I don't know, Mum,' he answered softly. No longer angry. 'I'm so tired.'

'I know. I know, love, but just hang in there, Josh. You are not alone. You are not alone, darling. We are right here. We are always right here.' I did my best to keep my tears at bay, knowing it would not help the situation.

We kept him on the phone, talking softly, talking rubbish, he barely responded:

'It was very frosty this morning . . .'

'I have been writing today . . .'

'We popped in to see Nanny and Grandad . . .'

'Did you have some lunch . . .'

'Simeon has been in the garden . . .'

'Ben is in Liverpool . . .'

Anything to pass the minutes while we caught red lights and sat in traffic that was maddening, until eventually, thankfully, we pulled up outside his halls of residence. I hung up and Simeon called Josh from his phone, thinking that a less emotional intervention might be the best thing. I found this galling as I was really trying, but had to remind myself this was not about me, it was about Josh and doing whatever necessary. But I so wanted to be the one with the answers.

'We are outside and we are not going anywhere, Josh,' I heard Simeon say. 'So even if we are here all night long. That's fine.'

We were walking the fine line between taking away the small amount of control he had over his life and his future and the desperate need to barge down his door, scoop him up and bring him home. Simeon kept him talking and I left the car and phoned a well-known mental health charity who give out a helpline to call if you think someone might be in danger. I was at my wits' end and it took me several attempts to correctly identify and call the number, I kept misdialling, pressing the wrong option button or accidentally ending the call. I felt desperate and nauseous.

Eventually, I spoke to a man who suggested I call the police.

I tried to explain, my voice shaky, 'I think calling the police might inflame an already delicate situation. I just want some advice, what should I do? We don't know how to handle this or what to say for the best,' I gabbled. 'It feels delicate, needs careful handling and we are really struggling to know how best to help him.'

The man spoke in a very matter-of-fact tone: 'If your son is going to kill himself, try and make sure he does so without causing danger or harm to others. And call the police.'

I hung up. I wanted to rant at him, to swear!

It wasn't his fault. Of course it wasn't. What I wanted from the helpline was the panacea; the words of the magical spell to utter that would take us out of this nightmare. I wanted to know where to find the fairy dust to sprinkle that would make Josh well, would put Simeon and me back in the kitchen at home where we had been about to eat supper, laughing, before the call came in. The fairy dust that would mean I wasn't standing on The Downs in Bristol, in the dark, wearing my pyjamas and walking boots with tear-smudged make-up running down my cheeks, listening to my

husband whisper as though talking to a child. I remember thinking: *How much more of this can we take? How much more?* And then
instantly I pictured Josh's face, pale and struggling, and I felt like
rubbish; how dare I have those thoughts, this was what unconditional love meant: loving someone even when it's hard to love them.

I got back in the car and Simeon took my hand.

'This will pass, Josh. It will all be okay. It will *all* be okay . . .'

'I'm just . . . I've had enough.' Josh now fell silent.

That was it. Our cue to 'Go! Go! Go!'

We decided to take matters into our own hands. Josh might
have been a grown-up in the eyes of the law, but he was our child
and we let our hearts do the talking and instinct guide our actions.

Simeon gripped the phone and I could see he was very emotional, his voice cracked.

'We are taking you home, Josh.' He spoke firmly and I cried
as quietly as I was able.

'I can't . . . I don't want to,' came his weak and half-hearted
response.

'Josh! Listen to me. We love you and tonight this is not your
choice to make. We just need to keep you safe and we are taking
you home. Now, are you coming out or do we come in?' Simeon
held firm with a resolve that I knew I could not have matched, his
tone commanding and yet kind. In that moment there was no difference of opinion, we worked as our best, a team, and I was never
more grateful for his presence.

There was silence on the end of the line until eventually Josh
spoke.

'I'm coming out now,' he whispered.

Minutes later he walked into view. His head was hanging forward and he was in his pyjamas. He looked bowed, walked slowly,
but all I felt was deep, deep relief. Simeon lowered the phone and
let out a long sigh, as if he had been holding his breath. None of

us said a word as we bundled him into the car and drove home in near silence.

I felt my breathing return to normal and looked out of the window as I cried, silently. Josh in the backseat found it hard to stay awake, his head lolling to one side as Simeon navigated the busy roads home. I thought about when Josh was a baby and would fall asleep in the car on the way home from a day out or a family dinner. I would park the car close to our little basement flat in Clifton and lift him carefully from his car seat, resting his head on my shoulder and with his little legs dangling either side of my hip. Often I was reluctant, once inside, to put him into his bed, not when the weight of him in my arms and the trusting abandonment with which he slept felt so glorious. Sometimes, I would sit in the wide armchair by the window with Josh asleep on my chest and I'd watch the night sky through the panes of glass and feel like the luckiest woman alive. I didn't have much money. I was alone, lonely at times, I guess, working harder than was comfortable and yet in those moments with my child in my arms and the moon peeking through the bruise of clouds that hung in the darkening sky, I felt like I had everything. I *did* have everything and at that moment I wished I could rewind to then. I don't know why, maybe because I wanted a break from the constant worry of Josh's illness, and also at some level I think I believed that with another chance I would do things differently . . . What, I'm not sure: work less, play with him more, be more attentive . . .

Simeon pulled up outside the house and quietly woke Josh, who said nothing but walked in and climbed the stairs, one at a time as though it was Everest, each step followed by a moment to catch his breath and to ready his body for the next step. It was painful to watch.

That night we slept with the bedroom doors open like we used to so we could monitor him throughout the night. Well, I say slept, we lay quietly, too alert to sleep. Simeon and I held hands across the mattress and I was happy to see the sun. We had made it; one more night and one more day with Josh on the planet. My relief, however, was tinged with desolation. This was a major setback. I think Simeon and I knew at that point that university was a step too far for Josh. It was more than he could cope with. He wasn't ready. And no amount of new friends and change of scenery could offset the inevitable. I recalled my words of encouragement, spoken when he got offered the place at Bristol: 'This might be the fresh start you need! You can do it, Joshy! It might be wonderful!'

And then the very worst thought struck me: had I pushed him to accept the place? Was I one of the mealy-mouthed idiots suggesting he pick up the bloody box? *Just a tiny one . . . have a go . . .* when all he really wanted to do was climb into his bed-island refuge? I hated the idea. Had he accepted the place to please us? Had I let him down? I thought about the lunch we had taken him on before the start of the new term, the car chock-full of all the things he might need for his next adventure at Bristol and I remembered him leaving the table and going into the loo to throw up. I pictured his clammy hands, his manifest anxiety.

I crept along the hallway and looked at my boy who was again coiled in the middle of the mattress and I wept.

He stayed there for a week. It was a terrible week. Simeon and I were tired and snapped at each other and I wasn't very strong. In between radio interviews for my latest novel and a spot on a panel show for TV, I cried and cried. I was weary and defeated. Where did we go from here? Simeon and I chased the topic around and around coming no nearer to a solution. He was starting to lose patience and I was losing energy, a bad combination for us all.

Then one day, Josh appeared downstairs and just like that said he wanted to go back to university. Simeon and I were as cautious as we were fearful, keen to encourage his enthusiasm for leaving the bedroom, but equally wary of how quickly and how far he might fall. This felt like a huge leap from bedroom back to university life and one we worried was too much.

I remember he chatted in the car quite amiably, asking about my latest book and how it was going, and talking about how great it would be to finally move into the farm, and when that might happen. It was as if the terrible events of the previous Friday night had not occurred. But rather than worry, I took comfort from his 'normality' hoping, as ever, that this might be a turning point. Simeon and I shared a knowing, hopeful smile and my heart lifted. It was like living on a merry-go-round with the same markers flashing by on an endless cycle, but we didn't know how to stop it moving and couldn't have got off even if we wanted to, not with Josh glued to it.

There were so many turning points, so many false dawns when I thought we were on the right path to recovery. And these moments were glorious. The truth, however, was that no sooner had I breathed a sigh of relief and given thanks to the many and varied gods littering the surfaces of my home, that I would step around the next bend and find myself once again staring at a cliff edge where Josh was dangling by his fingertips.

The house was quiet and we ate supper just the two of us. It was nice to be alone and reflect on the last week. We were a little giddy, I think it was relief, but I remember we laughed a lot at stupid things. We also spoke about the book I was writing and what Simeon was up to at work. These small vignettes of normality were a mental holiday from the angst that dominated our lives. We watched some crap TV, snuggled together on the sofa, before falling into bed, exhausted as ever and asleep almost before our heads hit the pillows. I remember feeling quite happy.

The phone rang at 3 a.m.

I woke to find Simeon sitting on the edge of the bed and caught the tail end of the conversation.

'I'm on my way! I'm coming now . . .' He spoke groggily with the phone under his chin as he scrabbled on the floor for his jeans and car keys.

'What's happened? What's going on?' I switched on the lamp.

'Josh' – he swallowed and my heart sank – 'Josh is in A&E – he's . . . he's had an accident.'

'What kind of accident?' I hardly dared ask, my voice was small and I couldn't get a full breath. A car? A fall? An injury? My thoughts raced . . .

'He has hurt his wrist.' He nodded. We locked eyes and I knew it wasn't an accident. Simeon looked tense, tired and angry.

'I'll come with you.'

'No, Mand, stay here. I'll be as quick as I can. I promise.'

And just like that he raced down the stairs and disappeared out into the cold, dark night and I looked at the space in the warm bed in which he had been soundly sleeping only minutes earlier. I couldn't sleep, couldn't cry, couldn't do anything. I was numb. I was desperately worried about Josh, but also wondered what Simeon was thinking as he drove through the dark in the dead of night. I wondered if he was regretting hitching his wagon to mine and making our little family of four. Who could have bargained for this?

I went downstairs and sat by the window in my nightdress with a blanket over my legs, staring out into the darkness, waiting to see the headlights sweep up the road, bringing our boy and my husband home.

Three hours later as the day began to peep its head over the dark blind of night, the car pulled up. I rushed to the front door and ushered Josh in with Simeon following behind.

Josh looked deathly pale, his eyes sunken. His wrist tightly bound with a large white bandage snaking up his arm and over his hand. It was awful to see and my stomach was in knots. The bandage had a bright-red splat on it where his blood had soaked through. I felt sick.

'What happened?' I shook my head. He had been out of our care for a matter of hours and this!

'I . . . I fell into some, erm . . .'

'Some glass,' Simeon finished.

'Some glass? How on earth . . . Josh . . . What . . .' I was lost for words.

Simeon shook his head at me subtly.

'We can talk about it tomorrow.' His voice was gravelly.

I smiled, to try and hide my distress. 'I'll go make some tea.' It was what I did in any emergency, put the kettle on and made tea. It might not solve anything, but it was the distraction I needed to gather my thoughts.

I filled the kettle and flicked the switch, trying to sort my muddled head. What had he done? How had he done it? I felt sick with tiredness. It was then I heard a thump, as if someone had fallen. In fact, exactly as if someone had fallen.

Josh . . . I raced into the sitting room and will never forget the scene that greeted me.

It wasn't Josh who had collapsed, but Simeon.

My pillar of support, my rock, my foundation, my night-time hand-holder, my strong soldier was coiled on the carpet with his hands over his head, as his body heaved and he was sobbing.

Josh was in the chair I had only recently vacated.

I dropped to my knees and wrapped my arms around my man. I had no words and it was all I could think to do – to hold him tight. I cried too, for so many reasons, partly to see my man so distressed, but also because I knew this was a crossroads; he had had enough, we had had enough and what did this mean for the future of our little family?

And there we sat, on the floor with our distress raw. Sobbing, propping the other up, quite literally, as we got to the end of the line. We were broken, almost, and it had taken this final straw to make us see it.

'Simeon!' I sobbed, 'Simeon, please . . .' I didn't know what I was pleading for, didn't know what else to say. It felt like an eternity before our crying subsided. We sat up straight with our backs against the wall, facing Josh who sat in the chair in the window. He stared at us, holding his bound wrist in his good hand with his face contorted. Simeon and I held hands, dried our eyes and took deep breaths. We had done our best over the last couple of years to shield Josh from our distress, our exhaustion, thinking he had enough to cope with, but that ship had sailed, here we were laid bare and Josh was the witness.

'We can't do it anymore, Josh.' I spoke for us both. 'We know you are sick, but you have to try, you have to help us to help you.'

Josh nodded.

I felt a complexity of emotions: I was tired, yes, but also furious that we were in this position as well as desperate, desperate to help Josh get better. 'Everything we suggest, every single thing: like changing your diet, taking supplements, trying to get fit, meditation, walking, fresh air, getting a pet, therapists, residential care, hospitals, everything we suggest you say no, no, no! And we are out of ideas! We are out of ideas and we are exhausted.'

Again Josh nodded, as he cradled his bandaged wrist against his chest. It tore my heart to see him like this, he looked like a child and this only caused me to cry again. Simeon gripped my hand tightly and I remember looking out of the window at the streetlight and thinking how I might quite like to stand up, go out of the front door, close it behind me and disappear . . . Selfish, I know, but I was truly at my wits' end.

'I can't do it anymore, Josh. It's affecting everything and I don't know how to stop you hurting yourself and I feel like everything we do is just putting off the inevitable that you will one day kill yourself. It's like living on the edge of a cliff and I am constantly catching my breath waiting for you to tumble over the edge.'

Josh made a sudden noise.

A loud slow noise like an animal wounded.

He cried out and said, 'I didn't realise . . . You two are everything, I didn't realise . . .' His tears came quickly and ridiculously, bizarrely – I was happy! Because Josh was crying: a tangible, real emotion! Something! Tears from this statue of a boy who had carried the same blank expression for months now and who walked shakily through life like a robot who was out of juice. The noise he made and his tears reminded me, if ever I had needed it, that Josh, our vibrant, smart kid, was still in there somewhere and that really, really did feel like a turning point. I leaned over and held his hand and the three of us stayed like that, a triangle of distress, each trying to catch a break.

'You need to help us, Josh.' Simeon took up the mantle.

'I will.' He nodded. 'I will. I'm sorry.'

'You don't have to be sorry,' he assured him, 'you never have to be sorry, mate. We love you. We do, Joshy. Being ill is not your fault, but we need to make changes, we need you to try things, be open to things or we are all going to sink.'

'Yep, yes, I want to. I want to feel better,' he managed.

I don't know how long the three of us sat like that in relative silence, each offering up a quiet suggestion of how we could go forward, but I know that by the time we stood and made our way up the stairs to bed, it was a new day.

A brand-new day.

Simeon and I crawled under the covers and I lay staring at him. His eyes were swollen and his breathing irregular, that of someone not used to crying like that. His reaction had reminded me that he was human too and he was a human in need of support. I had been so lost in my own battle, trying to stay afloat, write books, appear on TV, talk on the radio, care for Josh and all the other vagaries of family life that I had forgotten that this man, my husband, who was also a dad, was suffering too. I resolved to listen to him more, as I reached across the mattress to take his hand. And this I vowed to continue to do, knowing the comfort it could bring at the end of a long, long day.

'I love you, Simeon.'

'And I love you always.'

And I believed him.

Chapter Twenty-Two

Josh

'The return of colour'

'I went away and drew up a list of all the things you wouldn't have to suffer if you weren't here anymore. It was something like this: no more illness, no struggling, no loss, no heartbreak, no ageing . . . But then I considered all the things you would not experience: knowing the blessing of a child, earning the right in old age to become eccentric, getting properly drunk on champagne, sleeping in a meadow, by a brook, waking wrapped in the arms of the one you love, fresh caught lobster eaten on a dock, laughing so hard at nothing much that you feel dizzy with happiness. Oh, my darling, this list is endless, it stretches on for infinity . . .

Amanda Prowse

The night I ended up in A&E was one of countless nights when I'm ashamed to say I was so drunk I blacked out. I had been out with my friends, drinking, and made my way back to the halls of residence. This level of drunkenness, to the point where I lost awareness, had happened a handful of times before, but this night the consequences of it were a lot worse than finding myself on the floor of my mates' bedroom still in my coat and clutching a kebab. I came to, for want of a better word, stumbling and alone in the shared kitchen and I had badly cut my wrist by shoving my arm through a glass window and dragging it down. It was pretty bad, a mess. It's actually quite hard to think about and even harder to write about. I know there was a large pool of blood on the floor. My arm hurt, but the alcohol numbed me to the worst of the effects. Half of me wanted to bleed out. The solution, I guess.

I hovered in the hallway, deciding whether to go and lie on my bed and let nature take its course or to seek help. As I considered this my friend Alex, who lived on the same corridor, appeared and took control. He was horrified, shocked by the sight of me and his expression told me how bad it was. I was too numb to properly take in what was happening and I don't remember much detail about the incident itself, but I do remember those who now gathered around me, panicking. I have been told since that a member of staff was called, took one look at my injury and nearly passed out.

I made it to A&E via a speeding Uber, the consensus being it would be quicker than waiting for an ambulance. Alex travelled with me, sitting alongside. He had wrapped my arm in a towel. On arrival at the hospital, I was rushed through. The medic removed shards of glass from the wound and they stitched me up before bandaging my wrist and arm. I had sobered a little by the time I called home and spoke to Simeon, who came to collect me. He was calm at the hospital and in the car he was quiet, and I was thankful, not wanting to have to elaborate on the night's events. I didn't want to discuss it, didn't want to admit it, didn't want to think about it, but then when we got home . . .

This is hard to write, but my parents went hysterical. Hysterical.

I think they saw this as the first proof that I was not better, not as fixed as they had hoped and not happy, not at all. I was a mess, a fucking mess, so what's new?

In the weeks preceding my trip to A&E, my old friend depression had been dragging me down. I had stopped going to lectures, stopped working, stopped engaging and had again taken to my bed. The one place I felt safe and where I wasn't going to be judged.

The night I arrived home with my arm and wrist heavily bandaged, changed things for me. It was the first time I saw Simeon upset – really, really upset. He kind of collapsed and it was hard to witness, knowing I was the cause. I don't like to think about it. I knew how much he had done for me and thought about the nights he had slept on my grotty bedroom floor, and to see him so at a loss for answers made me determined to do everything I could to try to find a way through the fog. I wanted to not let him down, didn't want to let my mum down, and the words she spoke really resonated. She said something about how they were out of ideas of how to help me or even what advice to give, and I realised that my depression was not only affecting me, it was affecting everyone. She also screamed that alcohol was not the answer. She was right. I needed to take control and at least try some of the things I had said no to before. I could see that I needed to make a change or we were all fucked. With hindsight, it's clear to me that this awareness of the effects of my illness on others was actually part of my recovery, something to which I had previously been either oblivious to or too mired in depression to care about. My parents' well-being and their interest in me didn't feel like a pressure, it felt like a concern.

The three of us sat in the lounge until it got light; I think Mum made tea, and by the time we climbed the stairs the atmosphere felt lighter, as if there had been a shift in our world, as if we were making progress.

I still have an ugly puckered scar that runs from the base of my hand up to the centre of my wrist. It aches in the cold and itches from time to time. I know my mum hates the sight of it, but I don't because it's a reminder of how vulnerable I was, of how far I have come, and also of that night when I climbed the stairs with a sense of determination and with the beginnings of belief that things could and would get better.

By this stage we had a date to move into our new home, a rural farmhouse, a place where there was space, light and peace. It is a haven for us all. I remember roaming around the land and feeling freer than I had in the longest time, as if it was somewhere I could breathe. We had only been in for about a week or so and Simeon and I were up in the paddock when out of the blue he said to me, 'Mandy and I have been thinking, how would you feel if you didn't have to go back to uni, not ever? If you never had to go to another lecture, if you didn't have a deadline, or an assignment or any prescribed reading and no exams. Imagine it, Josh, if you could leave the academic world and walk your own path, find your own way . . . How does that make you feel?'

I looked down over the fields that border the River Severn and a feeling came over me that was all-encompassing and which I can only describe as lightness. It was as if weights had been cut from ropes I had dragged behind me for the longest time.

I smiled at him and it was a new high and I think we all knew then that that was the answer. I would leave university. *I would leave university!* I would do something, anything, but it would be on my terms. It was a scary prospect, made easier by the support of my friends at university, who all said how they feared for me if I stayed. It was just before the start of our second year and I told the first of my friends over the phone. It felt like a big deal telling him I was leaving, but he showed none of the surprise I might have expected and said I should have left a long time ago. This group of mates and I are still very close, I see them most weekends and the fact that I'm at home and they are at university doesn't really come into it.

And that was it. It really was that simple. One or two emails later and I had left the environment that I had been working hard to gain entry to for the whole of my school life. In a matter of seconds I had done it. And it felt . . . it felt like it did on the afternoon you broke up from school for the summer holidays, or the best Friday night ever, knowing a long weekend stretched ahead. I was finally free, able to think about the future without the knot of dread in my stomach. And actually, I now *like* the idea of being a flag waver for an alternative way of life – university is not for everyone, no shit! And it does not have to be the goal. There are other paths.

University did not give me depression: nature did that. But depression is an illness that for me was exacerbated and poked into action by the pressure of university life, just like someone with the broken arm Mum spoke about trying to become a hammer thrower – it won't work. It can't. Because it's broken. Broken.

I now know I am ill-equipped to cope in an environment where, according to the *Guardian* in May 2019, 'Twelve students in Bristol have, or are suspected to have, killed themselves since September 2016.'[17]

At the time of writing it is sadly now thirteen: thirteen people just like me for whom life felt overwhelming. I feel very lucky to have been able to break free from it all and start over, shedding my skin.

Yet no matter how freeing, making that decision was just the beginning. It was one thing to feel like I was standing on a new path and that the world was full of opportunities, but it required a dramatic change in mindset not only for me but for everyone around me. All my life 'clever old Josh' had been led to believe that he was going to get a piece of paper that would tell the world how smart he was. He would work hard and gather a clutch of degrees to his chest, shoulder-barging his way through the world, carving his own path to greatness. And yet here I was. Starting over without the first clue as to what this newfound freedom might mean and what I was actually going to do with it. It was the first time since I was three years old that I had been outside of an academic establishment. It was a bit like being in free fall: scary but exhilarating. I was anxious about telling my nan and grandad. I felt like I was letting them down in some way, but they could not have been more supportive.

'We just want you to be happy, Joshy. That's all we have ever wanted . . .'

My relief was instant. I still found it difficult to tell strangers and acquaintances, who would say, 'Oh, you're at Bristol, aren't you, how's it going?' I would change the subject and be evasive, as if not quite ready to let the world know and still feeling that it was in some way a failure.

But not now. Now I say, 'It didn't work out for me. I left. I'm going to try something different. It was actually really bad for my mental health.' And interestingly, as soon I say this, they more often than not tell me the story of a daughter/son/brother/friend/neighbour/cousin/partner who didn't finish their course and who very often also had mental health issues. They tend to finish with the phrase: 'And it was the best thing they ever did . . .'

I find it sad that it is highly unlikely that this personal information, this insight into what is so common, would have been offered if I had not started the dialogue.

So with the decision made I moved back home and things started to get a bit better. The first and most important change was that I revised my diet and have lost a little over 30kg – yes, the physical benefits of weight loss are great: I look and feel better, but

231

mentally I think I now also understand that with my disposition it is far better to give my body good fuel rather than the fat-laden crap that was so addictive but did nothing to help my sluggish mind and body. I rarely drink and if I do, it'll be a beer at a cricket match or BBQ and a glass of something in celebration, but the thought of binge-drinking until I lose consciousness? The thought actually disgusts me.

It would be nice if I could say my energy returned overnight or that I crawled into bed one night without the strength or inclination to turn off the bedside light and woke the next morning with the energy and motivation of an athlete, double high-fiving the beam at the bottom of the stairs and cartwheeling along the hallway, but no, this was not how it was.

It was more of a slow stretch, a gradual awakening; so gradual in fact that I barely noticed it at first. But then one day I realised I was a little more engaged, my focus better, I could hear and retain what people were saying as long as they were brief and this was how it continued. My eyes seemed to open more fully, as opposed to the half-lidded haze that had filtered my world for as long as I could remember. And when I realised what was happening it gave me the confidence to look for more positives, to try more, do more as it felt like everything was heading in the right direction.

I can only liken it to any physical injury when suddenly you realise that it doesn't hurt quite so much and you are not quite as preoccupied with it every minute of every day and the pain of it does not keep you awake all night. Normality creeps in until it is possible *not* to think about the injury at all. I am not quite there. But I'm getting closer. And I don't know if I will ever be able to ignore the illness that has taken up residence in part of my brain, but it is certainly a little better. Eased. I can live with it and it can live with me.

Oh, and something else happened, again very slowly, but it was the exact reverse of what had happened to the way I saw the world when I first became ill. Slowly, ever so slowly, colours started to reappear – I was no longer living in a black-and-white world with grey around the edges, but I could see the blue sea and sky, pinks, reds, golds and oranges in flower beds and out over the fields, the grass was green, and my future? Well, even that looked quite rosy. Not that I had specific plans, but it was enough that I could *not* see the endless nothingness stretching on for eternity. That was enough to make me look at life in a different way – this brilliant life! I am a boy between the hold of his illness and a future that is as yet unwritten, and that is exciting.

While writing this book, Mum asked me in detail for the first time about the pills I acquired that day back in November 2016, which I thought would be my very last – a topic we had both avoided up until this point and I get why. It's not easy for me to reflect on or for her to have to imagine. We have decided to write the transcript of that conversation.

This is it.

Word for word:

'I find it hard, Joshy, to think of you having those things in your possession.'

'Why are you crying?'

'Because I can't stand to think about it.'

'For God's sake, it was three years ago, Mum!'

'Not for me, Josh. For me it's today. It's every night before I close my eyes to go to sleep. I can't help it.'

'I don't know what I can say to that.'

'You don't have to say anything. It's just how it is for me.'

(Awkward pause . . .)

'So, come on, you can ask me anything and I promise to be one hundred per cent truthful with you.'

'Anything?'

'Yep, anything.'

'Who broke that lamp when you were little and Dad and I were out and you said a burglar had done it and run away?'

'Ben. Ben did it. He kicked it doing karate moves.'

(We both laugh.)

'Poor Ben, he's not here to defend himself! Okay, erm . . . I do want to ask you about that time, that day, when you . . .'

'Go ahead. But no more crying. I can't tell you how much it really, really pisses me off.'

'Okay, I'll try, but I can't promise. I guess what I want to ask you first is why you didn't take the pills the moment they arrived? And trust me I am thankful that you didn't, you know that, God, obviously!'

'I do know that. Erm . . . I don't know why I didn't. I guess it was the first time I'd felt in control for a very long time and I s'pose that might have been a positive feeling, knowing I had an option. Yeah, the fact that it was me in control. I told myself it was about timing, and I remember at some point thinking about who would find me and hoping it would be the postman because he looked like he had seen a bit more life and not the nice lady who cleaned the communal areas of the flats. God, that's awful, like it isn't going to totally fuck up whoever finds you. But yeah, I remember thinking I'd rather it was the postman than the cleaner, who was nice. I must have thought about how it would upset her.'

'Did you . . . did you think goodbye to me or to us in your mind? Did you think about us at all?'

(Long pause . . .)

'I know you want me to say that I did.'

'I don't necessarily, Joshy. I am just trying to picture it, imagine it. Sorry.'

'I seriously can't talk to you about this stuff if you keep breaking down. It's like it's too much.'

'It is too much! Jesus Christ, it is too much!'

'Okay, so no.' (Josh shakes his head.) 'I didn't think about you or Sim or Nan or Grandad or anyone, erm . . .'

'Well, apart from the cleaner and the postman.'

'Yep, weird when you put it like that. I don't even know their names.'

'Don't get me wrong. It's not that I wanted to know I was prevalent in your thoughts. This isn't about me. I guess I am more interested in what the anchors were that kept you present and, oh my God, I am so grateful to the lady who was nice and cleaned your hallways because it sounds like she might have been part of your reason to stay, even if you weren't aware of it.'

'A small part, yes, maybe. That sounds nuts.'

'Did you not think about H?'

'I think I thought about her after,' (H is my brilliant little sister, Hannah – from my dad's relationship with his partner, Emma) 'when I came home and when I was starting to feel a bit better – I used to think if she needed me or needed something then I had to be in better shape to help her. But to be honest, Mum, even if I did think about H I was too lost for it to make any difference or for it to push me towards making a different decision.'

(Mum nods)

'What do you think would have happened if fate had not intervened and you had been left alone with those tablets? Would you have taken them the next day or the day after that?'

'I can't possibly answer that, can I? I don't know.'

'So, with the benefit of hindsight, thinking about those of us who love you – and there are lots of us – do you think that had you succeeded your act would have been selfish? To cause that much hurt? To go without giving us the chance to help you? Or say goodbye?'

'I can see that some people would *think* that, but it wouldn't have been selfish because that suggests that I would have been

235

making a conscious decision in my right mind; doing it [ending my life] without caring about the effect of my actions on anyone else and it wasn't like that, not at all. I wasn't thinking straight. I couldn't think straight. I was in pain and at the same time numb. I would have done it in that fogged state almost like I wouldn't have known what I had done, if that makes any sense. Like when you are so drunk you do things and can't remember. Exactly like that, but I was sober. Why are you shaking your head?'

'The horror of it, Josh. Just at the horror of it.'

'God, Mum, why are you crying *again*?'

'I'm crying because I came close to losing you and I can't even think about it. I love you, Josh.'

'Stop with the crying! You promised.'

'I didn't promise. I only said I'd try not to.'

'Well try harder! For Fuck's sake!'

And actually this dialogue raises a good point. I am sure some of you will think that if I had been *serious* about suicide then I would have done it immediately, wouldn't I? And to you I would say that this is pretty much the whole point of the book – to say, I wanted to die on that day, but not necessarily the day that came after. And that's the message: no matter how bad you feel, how low, how sad, how broken, tomorrow is another day and you might feel differently, and so please, please hang on, just hang in there . . . give it time, give it one more day and then one more day and then one more . . . Please do that.

Chapter Twenty-Three

Amanda

'The hardest of conversations'

'Courage to me meant ploughing through that dull gray mist that comes down on life – not only overriding people and circumstances but overriding the bleakness of living. A sort of insistence on the value of life and the worth of transient things . . . My courage is faith – faith in the eternal resilience of me – that joy'll come back, and hope and spontaneity. And I feel that till it does, I've got to keep my lips shut and my chin high, and my eyes wide.'

F. Scott Fitzgerald

It became clear that in order to protect his mental health, it was best that Josh left university. Simeon and I discussed it and he told me that when he suggested it to Josh, it was as if he had given him a gift. He responded immediately, didn't have to think twice. He had no plan, but this dilemma, compared to battling his declining mental health, was nothing. It all happened very quickly. The decision was made and the letter written in haste – or at least that was what it felt like. The reality, I am sure, was that at some level he made the decision on the day he started, or tried to start, revising for his A levels. It sounds unbelievable, but it's absolutely true that after Josh had made the decision, on that very afternoon, I noticed the tension was gone a little from his shoulders, his walk was sharper, more purposeful, as if he was no longer shuffling, trying to put off 'arriving' at a place he did not want to go.

It was a good day. A really good day!

I have heard advice given to young students in the first overwhelming stages of university life that it will get better, easier, and that they will find their stride, and for many this is no doubt true, but not for Josh. For him it was too much, all too much.

DROPPED OUT.

GIVEN UP.

QUIT.

Are just some of the words I've heard others associate with his decision and it's this language that I feel is so detrimental to those who want to choose a different path but feel unable to, and it is language of which I am mindful. I absolutely abhor the words 'dropped out' when discussing students who leave their course. A 'university dropout' has such a negative connotation with suggestions of failure that can only add to the stress and feelings of negativity when someone who has every right to change direction or decide it's not for them makes the decision to leave. In many cases, Josh's included, it is actually one of the bravest things to do: bucking the trend; going against all that was expected or assumed, especially when that place was hard won; challenging the future they had been working towards. I much prefer to hear that they 'changed their mind', 'altered their life plan', 'left studying', 'picked a different path' . . . All much more hopeful!

I hate that for some students it feels easier to end their lives than to change course. What a terrible indictment of our society. And it's not only in the UK: an article published on the American website College Degree Search entitled 'Crisis on Campus' states '6 per cent of undergraduate students in four-year colleges have "seriously considered" attempting suicide in the past year. Nearly half did not tell anyone.'[18]

When they know they will be judged, it is hard enough for students to make the decision that might best suit their physical and mental well-being without having to justify it. And this is before we consider the debt some students incur, especially in the UK – debt that still looms large even if you have a change of heart. To be labelled a 'dropout' too feels unnecessarily antagonistic and a little cruel. Goodness, can you imagine if every time you changed a job, moved house or made a decision that you considered was for your betterment, you were labelled a 'dropout' or a 'quitter'? Flippin' 'eck! No wonder it's damaging to mental health!

I even had people say to me, 'Such a shame . . . a clever boy.' And, 'That's really sad.'

I have to bite my tongue and not point out the irony that it would be '*such a shame . . .*' and '*really sad*' if my son had stayed in that environment where he felt so ill that he might actually have succeeded in killing himself.

So yes, it was a good, good day. Not least of all because Josh came into the living room that evening smiling! And it was a proper 'showing his teeth' smile that I had not seen for a number of years. He placed his hand on his stomach where his anxiety liked to gather and he said, 'I feel a little bit excited.'

EXCITED! Oh my God, this one word, along with so many others, that had been missing from his vocabulary for the longest time. And they were missing because he had no need of them. Words like JOY, CONFIDENCE, OPTIMISM, HOPE,

POSITIVITY, MOTIVATED, ENERGISED and HAPPY – these emotions and feelings are the very opposite of depression. It felt like a massive breakthrough. No more than a first step, of course, but a first step that we had been willing him to take for years. We didn't expect him to break into a run anytime soon, but this day had been a long time coming and we celebrated it.

I realised that for years Josh had been trying to push his square mind into a round hole, an impossible and unpleasant, painful task, no matter that the task was padded with words of comfort, encouragement and support from all of us who loved him. Again with that glorious gift of hindsight, I can see that by trying to support and help him in the way we thought best, the way *I* thought best, it was possible that I was in fact clouding his thoughts when it came to making a decision, putting my positive spin on things.

You can do this, Josh!

We will help you in every way!

You are super smart!

Which I believe actually stopped him from being able to say sooner 'this is not for me' and walking away to pursue a path that gives him a better chance of mental health and that elusive happiness.

I feel the same about all the micro pressures that I have thrown daily in Josh's direction with the very best of intentions, and which he has confirmed were not easy to handle. Questions like: How are you? Are you feeling better? When do you think you might feel up to it? Questions that I used to think might help him focus, as well as wanting the answers myself – but I can now see they are the exact kind of question that add to the terrible burden of depression, weighing the sufferer down further when they really don't know how to answer.

So Josh was home, having made the decision to alter his course: not running around beaming, but there was definitely a lift in his mood. He started to eat right, paying particular attention to foods with too much sugar or certain fats and opting instead for a portion of protein and a mountain of vegetables. He also swapped sugary carbonated drinks for water – fizzy bottled water became his staple. He started to communicate a little more, asking questions as if he actually cared about our lives, and responded to us with more than a nod or shake of his head, a vacant stare or a one-word grunt. He began taking part in everyday activities that previously would have been beyond him, things most of us take for granted, like taking a shower, making a cup of tea and doing laundry. It felt like every aspect of his life and demeanour were progressing.

Josh had been home for a couple of months when I went to Majorca with my parents for a long weekend and it was on our first night away that Simeon called while we were having dinner.

'Mandy, it's me, Josh is in A&E . . .'

He cut to the chase and my head swam and I felt like the ground was rushing up to swallow me before he finished the sentence. I pushed my feet on to the warm floor to stop from falling off my chair. Simeon continued, 'He was with his friends and they were apparently playing American Football. He banged his head and they think he might have mild concussion.'

I laughed loudly, drawing stares from other diners and my parents too. Simeon laughed and there we were again in different countries gripping our phones, but this time sharing a different kind of moment. Now, I understand that for most to hear your son might possibly be hurt would not be a cause for celebration, but for me – it was a moment of happiness. I was hugely relieved that his trip to A&E was not for something more sinister, but also the fact that he had spent time with his friends and was outside . . .

'Tell him he's an idiot!' I laughed.

'I will. And I love you.' Simeon was smiling, I could tell.

'I love you too.'

So here we are, nearly four years on from the point when things started to unravel for Josh, and indeed for us as a family. We have come through a lot, but we are still standing. Just.

Josh is not fixed.

Josh is not cured.

But he is alive and that is everything.

The fear that he might lose his battle has subsided a little – I sleep better, fret less – but it is still present. I was/am afraid of doing or saying the wrong thing and fearful that 'the wrong thing' might end up being the straw that breaks his back, the action or phrase that makes him jump, makes him swallow the pills, raise the blade.

For me, at its worst, it felt a lot like living on a knife-edge with a chasm either side, plus the knife was on fire, I was barefoot, bullets rained down, I couldn't breathe, there was an angry dragon circling overhead and no one could hear me call for help . . . Yep, that's what it felt like. But now? It's about the same, but I am wearing shoes, I know the bullets are blanks, I have tamed the dragon and I have found my voice. I can call for help, I CAN SHOUT LOUDLY!!!

And I intend to.

My experience of caring for Josh and having to explain his illness is one that has shaped the way I look at sufferers and those who care for them and I know that the smallest bit of understanding makes a whole world of difference. The irony isn't lost on me that the negative and disbelieving reactions of many are the very worst thing for someone whose brain is already surfing on a sea of chaos and self-doubt to have to cope with. I guess the message is that it can happen to anyone. It can happen to someone you love and it can happen to you and we should all think about that.

When I read the all-too-familiar and heart-wrenching story of another young person who has died too soon, I feel a sickness come over me. I think about the unimaginable turmoil that person must have felt if suicide felt like the only or best option, but also I think about their mum, their dad, their siblings, friends and those close to them and I wonder what they were doing at the time they died. I think about the parents who held a small, wrapped parcel of newborn in their arms just like I did and who no doubt murmured the same wishes, hopes and dreams for all that their child might grow up to be . . .

And my heart flies across the miles to them.

And the reason I wonder what the people close to these sufferers were doing at that precise moment of demise is because I know that there have been times when it was nearly 'that day' and 'that moment' for me.

Since talking publicly about the writing of this book and about my son's depression I have received messages from students themselves who really, I think, just wanted someone to talk to, and my heart breaks for each and every one of them. They talk about the pressure, the stress, the desolation and the exhaustion and the fact that their parents either don't understand the pressure they are under, often believing the hype that student life is one long party! Or, they don't want to let their parents down, aware of their support both emotional and financial, as well as their expectations. They talk about the fast-paced, ever-changing world and one student described his situation:

'It's like you compare notes against everyone you meet, socially, academically, in every way. You look at what they have achieved and wonder how you would fare against them if you were both competing for a job . . .'

I found this unspeakably sad. I am in my fifties and a degree for my peers was almost a guarantee of a job, maybe not the job you really wanted, but a job. Now? Every CV is bursting with fantastic grades and extracurricular activities like playing an instrument, speaking four languages and juggling chainsaws while on a unicycle – all of this with the need to look perfect on social media – sweet Lord above! Is it any wonder they are so stressed!

And another student told me, 'It's like I'm here, but I am not here. I am going through the motions, but I don't feel part of it. I told my dad, but he said I was lucky: my sister is a nurse and she works long hours for low pay. He didn't get it. I don't know what to do next . . .'

I wanted to drive to the other end of the country and scoop her up.

I think it is vital that we try and demystify, unclutter and untangle the thorny web of depression and what it feels like to reach the point of suicide. We need as a nation, as parents, as carers and as educators to take a step back and ask what we really want for our kids, because driving them to succeed in this competitive, unforgiving, judgemental world could possibly cost them their happiness or worse . . .

I hope our honest, open account sends a message for any young people who are in the grip of their illness and who might be considering suicide. And I hope it gives some direction for those who love them. I have made a lot of mistakes – I was blinkered, but I have learned that it's not always best to go straight into solution mode. Sometimes there is no solution and therefore it's not always better to do 'something'. Sometimes all I need to do is listen and be calm. I have also learned that we need to make the hardest of conversations easier to have. We need to remove the embarrassment and awkwardness around the topic and we need to be unafraid to ask, 'Are you feeling suicidal? Do you think you might want to kill yourself today?' Questions that are direct and can be answered with a 'yes' or 'no' answer. Allowing help or intervention to be immediate. It is also not a question about progress or choice, nor the kind of question that requires too much thought for a foggy brain, which can also feel like pressure: 'How are you feeling?' is hard for a sufferer to voice when they can't explain it even to themselves.

'Are you feeling suicidal?' This very question, so easy to write, easy to read, but so, so much harder to say out loud to the person you love when you know they are fragile. This I understand. I used to be afraid of it. But talking about it to someone, *anyone*, is key to immediate prevention. It's about trying to get sufferers through the dark times when the urge is strongest, because as Josh says:

'Things can and usually do get better.'

Simeon and I are both painfully aware that for the want of an hour or two or a different split-second decision, Josh would not be here and we are not about to waste this wonderful gift of a second chance. Yes, Josh gets better and stronger with each passing day, but we still keep him close, for now. His room at the farm will always be his safe space where he can retreat as and when he feels the need, a place to be at peace with his two beloved dogs when the world feels a little too much. And those days still happen. Josh is now so in tune with his depression that he looks for his signs, triggers, and we do the same. I also know that it's vital to give myself time and to remind myself not to feel guilty if I have a good day or a very good day. Josh's depression should not always cloak me.

If I try and look for the silver lining in this whole awful journey, I think there are a few. I certainly feel very close to Josh, like I know him back to front and inside out. And I treasure him. We have seen him at his worst and he us, and that makes for a deep bond, which I believe can only make us all closer. I think we as a family have a strong sense of what is important and we know that happiness does not lie in stuff, but in the small things, like a good night's sleep, a warm bath, a decent cup of tea.

Simeon and I are also solid as a couple, having had to work as a tag team supporting Josh for the last few years. Not that it has been easy and there were certainly moments when the relentless fatigue of caring for and about Josh was so wearing that I wondered if we would make it. They say what doesn't break you makes you stronger and I guess that's where we are. I value Simeon as a partner to me, supporting me in my darkest times, and as a dad to Josh – to whom he has devoted more sleepless nights and more hours of attention than anyone has the right to ask for.

I know that this support will be ongoing, but with Josh meeting us halfway and as the fog of his depression clears it doesn't feel like a chore, not at all. We are so very proud of him. So very proud of both our boys.

People *still* don't fully comprehend our son's illness, often asking:

'Why doesn't he get a proper job?'

'Is he asleep *again*?'

'Cheer up, mate, worse things happen at sea!!!'

This tone prevails because like it or not this is the reality of living with a mental illness. I wish people could spend a day, in fact just an hour inside Josh's head so they could, if not empathise, then at least understand.

And human to human I think that is all we can really ask for, isn't it? Understanding.

Time is a funny thing. It certainly moves faster the older you get and sometimes I sit and look in the mirror with more years behind me than ahead and it feels like only a year or so ago that I gave birth to Josh. I half expect him to waddle into the room gripping a dinosaur in his little fist with a nappy sitting slackly on his bottom and a gummy smile just for me. I hear the door open and look at the reflection of my son in the mirror, a man now, and I know that visually, had I been able to see this adult version of my small child I would have recognised him. But when I think back over the last few years to how Josh looked during the height of his depression: the hollow stare of someone who has had the marrow drawn from deep within and whose happy has fled . . . no, that person I would not have recognised. It would have seemed unfeasible, impossible and more frightening than anything I could have imagined.

I did in darker moments of self-doubt when he was small, sometimes ponder how I would cope if Josh ever got hurt, injured or became ill. The imagery that filled my head on those occasions was of my son in a hospital bed, wires and tubes attached, possibly sleeping, and with me in a chair doing my best to rally his spirits. Had someone told me that in just a couple of decades the thing that would be missing, lopped off, taken from him was his sparkle, his drive, his energy and his will to exist, well, that would have left me speechless and the questions, I'm sure, would be the very same ones that rattled around my head when his illness first struck.

I will admit, I have often wished to turn back the clock to do things differently, still at some level believing that there is something I could change that would effect a different outcome for Josh. And then I think: what would I change? And again I come unstuck. I would of course do the exact same things, not aware that anything needed altering and believing that I was doing the very best job of being a mum.

Josh is kind and has always displayed kindness. As a small boy he could not bear to witness injustice of any kind and was not averse to standing up and speaking his mind, no matter that the perceived injustice was being meted out by a person in authority like a teacher or indeed a much bigger, older boy.

I can see him now across the dinner table with me questioning him.

'Why did you even get involved, Joshy?'

'Because it wasn't fair, Mum! It wasn't fair.'

Josh taught me very early on a lesson that has served me well over the last few years: that sometimes it is necessary to do the right thing rather than the easy thing.

I now question whether this was down to the fact that he was often a victim of injustice himself, singled out for reasons beyond his control: dyslexia and an inability to catch a ball or run fast when such things mattered to those giving the lesson. It seems he was often unable to articulate what felt unfair about his own life but was quick and ready to do so for others. These foundations were laid early and I believe that it is at Primary education level that the conversation around mental health and identifying vulnerable children should begin. To be able to offer support and stop the escalation of depression can only be a good thing for the individual, as well as their families and communities. 'One in eight children have a diagnosable mental health disorder – that's roughly three children in every classroom' – a sobering statistic.[19]

I am a very different person to Josh and I'm usually happy, brushing off any dusting or hint of depression that dares land on my shoulders. My happiness, my upbeat persona seems to have been pre-programmed, nauseatingly so if you ask my peers and family who encounter me in the early morning when I smile at the day and prepare myself for all that it might bring – yes, apparently at those times my enthusiasm for life is nothing short of irritating. I think it's fair to say that my joyful disposition has not only made it harder for me to understand Josh's state of mind, but I suspect has for him been an unwanted comparison, magnifying something that has proved elusive. I genuinely try to keep a positive outlook – almost as if there is a balance that can be reached – and if Josh is feeling down or has a low mood, I can achieve some kind of equilibrium in the house by staying motivated and up. This is not always possible and very often his mood is like a sledgehammer to the sunniest of thoughts and moments. This can't be easy for him either although I'm sure that very often he is unaware of it.

Like the time we went to Florida. The holiday was wonderful, but not for Josh. I know he tried – tried to join in, tried to show enthusiasm – but with the bruise of fatigue sitting beneath his eyes and very little to offer by way of conversation around the noisy dinner table, I knew he wished he were anywhere else and that was heartbreaking.

I thought I was doing a good thing, giving him a treat, but instead it felt like I had handed him a two-week sentence and that was tough. It brought us all down.

We went to Disneyland for the day. I walked behind him, staring at the slope of his shoulders, his reluctance to walk, each step seemingly heavier than the last, and I knew all he wanted was to sleep. There was something about seeing him so down and withdrawn at Disneyland, where everyone was walking around with a perma-grin and having the very best time, that was grotesque and distressing in equal measure. He looked like the only sad face in a sea of happy and I thought it the perfect metaphor for my boy and my heart wept for him.

For Josh, on bad days, it feels like it is a combination of severe fatigue and the yoke of depression, which lasso the joy from the air and leave us all struggling under the oppressive weight of the atmosphere. I find these days difficult. But, thankfully, they are getting fewer and I only have to glance at the angry puckered scar on his left wrist to remember how far we have come.

I was in a car, travelling across Bristol with Josh about a year ago and I thought back to that time when he was little and we were heading to nursery, nearly twenty years ago now. The main difference being that on this day Josh was driving, I was in the passenger seat and he now had a beard.

'I remember, Josh, when you were little saying that you'd like to cut the grass on The Downs.' I laughed.

'I remember saying that!'

'And can you remember why you wanted to do that?' I asked.

I thought of how I had been full of disappointment as he dismissed my own suggestions of what his future self might achieve.

'Joshy! You can be anything you want to be! You are brilliant! Anything at all! A playwright or an astronaut exploring space! Think about it, wouldn't you like to climb a mountain or be a surgeon or play music?'

My grown-up son now looked out of the window at the tanned, laughing faces of the men riding the tractor-style mowers with trailers attached.

'Because they looked happy.'

'And now?'

He shrugged. 'I still think I'd like to do something like that.'

'Well, you can. You can do anything you want to.'

'I have been thinking . . .'

'Thinking what, Josh?'

'That I would quite like to tell people about my depression. Try and explain what it's like to live with it.'

'Okay, that would be brave and I guess my concern is that it would forever label you as the boy who has depression.'

'Mum, I *am* the boy who has depression whether I tell people about it or not.'

'I guess so. What are you thinking?'

'I could write a book.'

'Well, that would be a challenge for you with your dyslexia. How about we write a book together, it is our story after all?'

'No way. Firstly, it's *my* story and, secondly, I could never, ever, ever work with you on anything, ever. You'd drive me fucking crazy!'

'Actually, Josh, it's partly my story too, I did grow you after all.'

'No way, Mum! Absolutely no way. Forget it.'

Chapter Twenty-Four

Josh

'The endless path to happiness'

'Wisdom is oftentimes nearer when we stoop than when we soar.'

William Wordsworth

Depression is the vehicle that drove me to the brink of suicide and made me want to disappear from the face of the earth. I use the words easily and yet am fully aware of their connotation. It feels that getting the right treatment both physically and mentally is a bit of a lottery. In total, less than one per cent of the NHS budget is spent on children and young people's mental health services.[20]

In the US, 'It has been predicted that by the year 2020 total US expenditure on mental health services will reach some 238 billion dollars . . . Depression is one of the most common and well-known mental disorders. It is estimated that around 8 per cent of adults in the US suffer from depression.'[21]

Some people strike lucky and have doctors and mental health support within the stretched NHS that can make all the difference, others not so much, and this at a time when your thoughts are chaotic and the one thing you need more than ever is certainty, routine, a steady voice of reassurance and a strategy for living with the disease. I cannot imagine how horrific it would be to go through something like this without the support of a loving family, even if I didn't always want their love and intervention, and yet for countless people suffering – addicts, the homeless, the lonely and those who feel unable to ask for help – they feel entirely alone. Alone with the stigma, and crucially one step away from deleting themselves.

I think about it a lot, this suicide epidemic that is taking the lives of the young and is still on the rise. And it's kind of ironic that in a world of increased knife attacks, gun ownership and the many other perils the media highlights and which parents warn their kids about:

Don't talk to strangers!
Never accept lifts from someone you don't know!
Do not leave your drink unattended in a public place!
Take care if you walk home alone in the dark!
Don't do drugs!

the unbelievable and unpalatable truth is that the most likely person to murder you – is you!

Especially if you are young and male.

According to Health Profile for England 2018, looking at trends in mortality, in males aged ten to forty-nine years, suicide and injury or poisoning of undetermined intent is the greatest cause of mortality.[22] We have to try to stop this. More statistics are available at Mental Health UK.[23] 'The fact is suicide is the leading cause of death among young people aged twenty to thirty-four years in the UK and it is considerably higher in men, with around three times as many men dying as a result of suicide compared to women.'[24] And 'One reason that men are more likely to complete suicide may be because they are less likely than women to ask for help or talk about depressive or suicidal feelings. Recent statistics show that only 27 per cent of people who died by suicide between 2005 and 2015 had been in contact with mental health services in the year before they died.'[25]

The question as to why such a staggering number of young men are taking their own lives is a complex one and I know the answers are just as complicated. But here, in summary, are what I believe to be some of the contributing factors.

I feel comfortable in saying that most students don't feel wanted. The university culture in the UK in my experience is now one that is impersonal, an undergraduate sausage factory that takes the cash and neglects to learn about or invest in individuals. It is far from the movie ideal where students and professors gather for stimulating debate and an exchange of opinions in the quadrangle. In fact, it is far more like a business than a place of learning, where the teaching staff are pushed for time and pushed to get results and the students have very little contact with their professors other than attending lectures and the odd tutor group. It makes it hard to form relationships, which would go a long way to building stronger communities within faculties and therefore make the students feel like they belonged. For Freshers coming from the cosseted world of school this can be a shock, especially when for many this is their first experience of living away from home. For some, it must feel that all their stays of support have been cut simultaneously.

Speaking in 2017, student Lucia Villegas stated, 'Often, I feel overwhelmed. The demands of university work, having to take care of myself, social commitments and the general stress of living can pile on top of one another, until I can't see over it; like an insurmountable mountain sitting on my chest.'[26]

I know exactly what that feels like. And an article in the *Guardian* – 'You Are Not Alone' – detailed student stories of mental health. 'As a Fresher you are constantly reminded that this is supposed to be "the time of your life". When it feels like the worst time of your life you feel both a sense of guilt and a pressure to keep these negative thoughts to yourself.' And, 'I spent the first few weeks of uni hiding in my dorm room crying my eyes out. I was homesick and wasn't sure if I wanted to be there at all.'[27]

These sentiments are widespread. Student life can be wonderful, of course it can, the best time of your life. But it can also be isolating, with no real checks apart from buddy systems. There is often a short talk during Fresher's Week – an induction where attendance is optional – on how important it is to make everyone feel included and where helpline numbers are issued with the advice to call if anyone feels they are struggling. In my experience people with depression find it hard to ask for help, let alone call an anonymous helpline when they believe it will be pointless. These helplines are not always operated 24/7 and unsurprisingly many students reach crisis point outside of the regular nine-to-five of a working day. Also, they are sometimes run by volunteer students rather than professionals, and I question how well trained they are to spot the warning signs in a person whose mental health could be failing.

Finances are another factor. It has never been more expensive to be a student. Not only do students struggle to live in cities where the cost of living is high, but also there is the actual cost of attending university in terms of fees, etc. According to the *Financial Times* in January 2019, 'The average graduate in the UK from a three-year degree carries more than 50,000 pounds of debt and faces high interest rates.[28] The Destinations of Leavers From Higher

Education (DLHE) data reports £22,399 as the mean graduate starting salary with outliers excluded.[29]

And in the US The National Association of Colleges and Employers (NACE) calculates that the preliminary average starting salary for graduates from the class of 2018 is approximately $50,004.[30] According to *Forbes*: 25 February 2019 – 44.7 million students have student loans. The total US student loan debt is almost $1.5 trillion – making an average debt of $33,557 per student.[31]

This is an incredible pressure to put on young shoulders, a massive financial burden, especially when families have made sacrifices so their children can attend. It's a double-edged sword: large debt must be a great source of concern, but the fact that the debt is incurred whether you finish your degree or not, makes it so much harder to leave the course. Effectively you will have racked up that huge sum for nothing. Or at least it can feel that way.

Social media is, I think, one of the curses of our age. At a time of self-discovery, teens and twenty-somethings are under enormous pressure to look a certain way, live a certain lifestyle and even eat food that is Instagram-worthy! It is of course preposterous and that perfect life is nearly always unattainable. Most of us look and feel very different from these people who seem to have it all, and when you are suffering from depression or self-doubt, is it any wonder that – with the constant bombardment of a faultless yet unattainable standard, blasted into the palm of your hand every minute of every day – students suffer with low self-esteem and feelings of failure?

An *Independent* article entitled 'Six Ways Social Media Negatively Impacts Your Life' stated '. . . our reliance on social media can have a detrimental effect on our mental health. In March 2018 it was reported that more than a third of Generation Z [mid-1990s–mid-2000s] from a survey of 1,000 individuals stated that they were quitting social media for good, as 41 per cent stated that social media platforms make them feel anxious, sad or depressed.'[32]

Plus there is, I believe, an unrealistic expectation of what university life will be like. We are the fame generation, weaned on reality TV and competitions where the goal is to get through to the next round and the next and the next and where being famous/popular/gaining 'likes' is currency. The truth is it is actually hard to achieve any level of popularity and yet for many this feels like the goal. University is lauded as the time of your life and for those who are not invited or do not have a large friendship group, who are possibly feeling the chill of loneliness, it can be exacerbated by the belief that everyone else is at a party, and one to which you are not invited.

We are also the generation who talk more and communicate less. We have the need to be constantly connected, updated, plugged in and we gaze at screens, often lacking in skills for the face-to-face stuff. When you are an anonymous user sitting behind a keyboard you can be anything you want to be and coming clean about feeling sad, scared or suicidal is, unsurprisingly, not high on the list of what impresses. Not only must these interactions feel unfulfilling, but it is hard when you are out of the habit to take off the mask when face to face, hard to be open when you do not have the experience or the confidence to be so.

Life can feel very much like a race where there is little room for kindness or for niceness, not when there is so much intra competition to be the best of the best, to win a place at university, gain a first, get a job, beat all other applicants, climb on to the housing ladder (if you are very lucky), make money, have a perfect relationship, travel the world, make more money and be a winner, whilst not forgetting to show your altruism in the form of charity, and your beauty captured in any number of selfies with interesting or exotic backgrounds!

Among my peers I have seen their anguish at having to admit they have failed a subject or a module, dropped a grade or done less well than expected: not the end of the world of course, but it can sure feel like it. University culture where each person is reduced to a candidate number and a set of grades makes it very hard to admit failure. How often do we hear the phrase 'Failure is not an option!' but in my opinion failure *should* be an option. Accepting failure should be encouraged as a way to learn from mistakes, turning students into rounded citizens rather than anxiety-ridden or depressed ones. I prefer the idea that it's better to try and to fail than not to try at all. In the science community, 'failing' or 'changing the plan' is exactly how we learn what doesn't work, taking us one step closer to discovering what does. I like this.

In almost every aspect of student life we are trying to win – to be perfect. Is it any wonder then that when it feels like you are *not* going to win, in fact not even going to finish in the top ten, it might seem easier to check yourself out of the race altogether?

There is also a distinct dislike of averageness. Everyone is told they *can* be great, all they have to do is wear the right brand, drive the right car, listen to the right music on the right device, go to the right clubs, get the right girl/boy and earn the right amount of money – and so it is quite unsurprising that if you don't meet these ideals you plummet. We need to recalibrate what constitutes success, as currently I feel there is no scale and often no truth – I would have fared better if I'd known it was okay to fail and be average – but again, no one puts the truth on social media. You are effectively comparing your mundane life to other people's highlight reels.

And finally, I feel that suicide is on the rise because the more young people end their own lives, the more young people *will* end their own lives. This feels particularly poignant to me as a former student at Bristol University, where it is suspected that between 2016 and 2019 thirteen students killed themselves.[33] And I think there is real danger to the young and vulnerable when a large number of students have died by suicide as it somehow normalises the behaviour.

I fear for that groupthink mentality. I have watched with interest the protests from students at the University of Bristol against the cuts in mental health services and pastoral care in the halls of residence. Ruth Day, who helped organise a march in protest at the University's health crisis, said services were 'still badly overstretched' and that the march was organised by a collective of university societies who felt services were still 'inaccessible . . . When you get to access them they are fantastic but there are so many people with problems and they are having to wait as long as five weeks to be seen – these people may not be suicidal at the start but they are at risk.'[34]

My personal journey in and out of hell has lasted about six years. And whilst I am not free of depression and accept that maybe I never will be, I can now see a road ahead; or maybe it's more accurate to say that I can see a bend in the road ahead, although I can't see what lies beyond it. Believe it or not, this is a positive thing because previously I could only see the long, straight eternal road to nothingness. This bend in the road that has appeared now presents an opportunity. And around that curve lurks the tiniest possibility of something different, a new feeling, an altered state and for now that's enough – I can *see* the bend whereas at the height of my illness I couldn't even see tomorrow.

For me, living with depression is exactly the same as accepting any other long-term health condition. I will do my best to manage it, stay one step ahead of whatever it throws in my path, but ultimately I suspect it ain't going nowhere!

I don't like what I am going to say next, I am not proud of it, but I think it's important.

It's important to me.

And it's the truth.

I have a confession, a terrible confession and it is this: prior to getting ill, I never believed anyone with depression.

I didn't think it was real.

There. I've said it.

I thought depression and feeling a bit fed up were about the same thing. I suspected one person's depression might be another's disappointment and I also thought it might be code for 'too lazy to do . . . anything'.

The term depression was, to me, no more than an umbrella excuse and the reality is I have heard this belief shared by many.

I would like to say I am sorry. I apologise for my lack of understanding and I wish that my assumptions had been true, because that would be far preferable than the reality of the illness that almost stole my life.

I therefore knew with certainty that when *I* used the word 'depression' there would be a swathe of people who would be thinking as I used to:

'Just get on with it.'

'How weak.'

'What have you got to be depressed about?'

'Man up!' – I hate this phrase so much. For me it's indicative of toxic masculinity that harks back to the days of old when men had stiff upper lips and women were the emotional beings. Thank fuck we have moved on. Well, most of us, but there is still a long, long way to go. I think if men and boys were less concerned with 'manning-up' and were more honest about how they were feeling, if they could reach out, openly and honestly without fear of ridicule or feeling that to show emotion was in some way emasculating, then quite possibly the depression and suicide rates among young men would not be rising.

And even on days when my depression seems to be at bay I live with the permanent and lingering scent of shame that is associated with the condition. I am ashamed of the state of my mind, even though I am aware that there is nothing I did to cause it and nothing I could have done to prevent it taking hold, it is just how it is. I think the shame is something I will always carry and it is largely down to how I know society generally thinks of mental illness. Like a bad smell that no matter how many people tell me is fine, undetectable, I am aware is right there under my nose and under theirs too. It's horrible.

I am putting my innermost feelings on the pages of this book for you to see. And trust me, for someone who found it hard to buy a ticket on a bus or order a drink in a coffee shop, this has been no easy task, but I want to join the movement of men and boys who are starting to say, 'I cry', 'I suffer' and sometimes 'I need a bit of support'. So check on your friends, ask your team mates, invite the people who are quiet and keep an eye on those who might be the life and soul, but who you know are painting on a mask – we need to keep the conversation going, one with mental health at the centre of the discussion.

I like the phrase: 'Be the change you want to see in the world.' This really strikes a chord with me. I am doing my best to be open about the way I feel, about my emotions and about my illness, because one thing is for certain: we need to change things.

I need to change things.

Knowing the general consensus on depression greatly affected my need for isolation because I knew what non-sufferers were thinking, even if they didn't say it out loud. This knowledge added to my loneliness and was an unfair and unnecessary burden on top of everything else. To anyone who still has these thoughts, who believes that depression is a myth or can be shrugged off, fixed with no more than a good night out or by simply 'pulling yourself together' I would say this:

Depression came along like a wall of water that knocked me off my feet. I didn't see it coming; I wasn't expecting it, I thought I was on solid ground. Each time a wave hit, I scrabbled to my feet, only for another wave, larger than the first, to smack me back down to the ground. It was exhausting and relentless. Everyone can survive the first couple of waves but when you have lost count and you are tired it takes more than most people know to get back up.

If it can happen to me it can happen to you, and a little kindness and understanding goes a long, long way. But in some ways I am *glad* if you don't understand depression because it means you haven't experienced it and I wouldn't wish for *you* or *anyone* to know how truly terrible and isolating it feels.

The reality is I took to my bed and spent the best part of three years taking medication, sleeping (a lot) and talking to various doctors and therapists, each visit leaving me more disillusioned and frustrated than the last – many didn't give a shit, didn't have time to give a shit and I could feel their sighs of irritation when I again recounted that I felt exactly the same as I had the last time I saw them – what did they expect? Star jumps and confetti? This was depression not a fucking cold! All they could do and all they did was put me on waiting lists, make the next appointment and write me a prescription for drugs. And that is just not good enough. Therapists were for me a bit hit and miss and psychiatry, the few times I attended, made a difference, but I was lucky. I am lucky.

Angry? Yes, I am angry – my family, grandparents, Mum and Simeon were the sticky tape that just about held me together, but not without personal cost. And what about the millions of people who don't have a Mum-and-Simeon safety net? What if they have GPs who are as shite as mine? What hope for them? I can imagine how they are feeling today, right now, and I hate that they feel that way. I want to say to them, to you, hang in there. Please, hang in there.

I hope I am encouraging the dialogue on depression and giving those who suffer a glimmer of hope because despite my illness I live a good life, a really good life! I find it sad that most people I meet are unwilling to share their own story, their own suffering, until they know of mine. I'm confident this personal information, this insight into what is so common, would not be offered if I had not started the dialogue and raised the topic, such is the extent of the stigma.

What brought me back from the brink were a few simple things that made all the difference and it is these few things that I want to share with you if ever life feels like too much:

- Try not to think too far ahead.
- Breathe. Take deep breaths and keep breathing.
- Don't panic, take things a minute at a time, an hour at a time, and each hour you get through is an achievement.
- Don't compare yourself to anyone else. Nothing and no one matters as much as your mental health and keeping you present. Right now.
- Drink water.
- Eat some food.
- Wash yourself.
- Keep warm.

And to those carers/guardians/friends looking after someone with depression, remember it's the simple things that make a big difference, just like with any physical illness:

- Make sure they have enough water or a cup of tea.
- Take them outside for air or open a window.
- Sit quietly with them and offer calm distractions if appropriate, give them good reasons to stay alive, things to hope for, remind them of the people who love them and the difference they make to their lives.
- Talk gently about the future – something tangible, an event, a day.
- Give messages of hope and positivity.
- Hold their hand.

It really is as simple as doing all the things you would do with any other sick person, because when you are in the grip of illness, mental or otherwise, it is often about the small stuff, fulfilling basic needs and taking baby steps that can be a turning point. There is nothing nicer than climbing into clean bed linen when your bed is your prison, and taking a shower can change the way you feel about yourself and your surroundings. These small acts of kindness and understanding are incredibly helpful for someone with depression.

Never forget, whether you are a sufferer or a carer, that you are not alone. There are millions of people going through the exact same experience at this precise moment in time. And it affects people from all walks of life. Lady Gaga, Hugh Laurie, Gwyneth Paltrow, Brad Pitt, J. K. Rowling, Eminem, Steven Fry, Alastair Campbell, Abraham Lincoln, Sigmund Freud, Winston Churchill, Franz Kafka, Mark Twain, Charles Dickens, Dwayne 'The Rock' Johnson, Ian Thorpe, Sir John Kirwan, Dan Carcillo – they have all suffered or suffer with depression. Every single one of them.

If you are reading this on a bus, train, tube or plane, in a classroom or coffee shop, a waiting room or a beach, just take a moment and look around you – who looks like they are suffering? Anyone? No one? Hard, isn't it, because sometimes those laughing the loudest could be the ones suffering the most. I really like this anonymous phrase I read: 'People who need help sometimes look a lot like people who do not need help.' I think it says it all.

Depression doesn't discriminate. It doesn't care about your race, creed, colour or sexuality; it doesn't care about your wealth, your poverty, your politics or your lifestyle. Depression can get its claws into you and once it does it's very hard to shake them off.

No one is immune.

The nature of depression means brain fog is the enemy of all logical suggestion – so the very things that those thinking clearly might suggest are often the very things that are hardest to grasp or comprehend.

Now things are different for me.

I might not always be able to control my illness, but I own it.

I state it without awkwardness or embarrassment to anyone who asks. It is not a badge or my defining characteristic, but it's part of me and, who knows, in the future, it might be no more than a footnote to a long and successful life, but the simple fact is: I have survived depression just like anyone survives a physical illness. The main *difference* is most people like me feel it's better not to mention it because whilst the topic is more freely discussed there is still a stigma attached.

WE NEED TO SMASH THE TABOO and REMOVE THE STIGMA!

I wish I could say my recovery has been quick, instant, but it hasn't. It isn't. It has in fact been a painfully slow process. My mental anguish did not disappear overnight and there was no flash-bang moment. For me, it has been like a slow reveal until one day I became aware of the gloom lifting and with that came the understanding that I did not feel quite as bad as I had.

One thing that is as fresh today as it was during the height of my depression is the guilt I feel. Guilt seems to be one of the many scars that still remain no matter how I try to justify my illness or am told by others that my guilt is misplaced. Maybe it will fade in time, who knows?

I still have physical limitations with my joints and I am prone to migraines, having suffered with them for the last couple of years, the reason for which is still elusive. When they come I lose my sight, my head feels like it has a cleaver in it and I throw up at the slightest exposure to noise or light. They can last for twenty-four hours. I hate it when one is looming because I know what I have to look forward to – and there isn't a thing I can do about it. I am not surprised I have migraines – I mean, why not? It's just another facet of my brain, just another way I feel my head is completely messed up!

Some of my anxieties still persist – I find some things extremely stressful, like new or unfamiliar situations, meeting strangers, one-to-one stuff – and I still absolutely hate opening emails and mail. I can't explain why, but I feel that whatever is waiting for me inside any message can only be bad and it is therefore best to avoid them at all costs. I didn't say it was logical.

I am glad to say I no longer live a horizontal life – one where I lie in bed looking at the ceiling – ticking off the seconds, the minutes, the hours and the days, wishing life would go faster or stop altogether. I am now integrated back into society (almost). I drive, and that freedom is a great feeling. I work and I am physically healthier than I ever have been. I have two French Bulldogs, Dottie and Beau, who are criminal masterminds, finding new and ingenious ways to keep me on my toes. I have energy and am motivated; excited to see what comes next. My path to recovery is a long and winding one and I think it might in fact have no destination, no end, but it is a path that has led me to sport, fitness, weight loss, the great outdoors, an obsession with music and the love of my two pups, to name but a few things. Life now feels more like an adventure and less like a chore and the fact that I can feel excitement about this or anything else is huge when not so long ago I was a living empty shell, numb and clinging to life with indifference.

I don't know what my future holds, who does?

But the fact is: I am still here. I am glad I came out the other side. I have made changes to my life and I did not disappear from the face of the earth.

I DID NOT TAKE MY LIFE.

I am, in fact, for the first time in as long as I can remember, on solid ground and here is where I hope to stay.

And so here I am, writing a book – who'd have thought that I, Josiah Hartley, would be capable of something like that?

Actually, me! *I* thought I was capable of something like that . . . I just got a bit sidetracked.

Depression will do that to you.

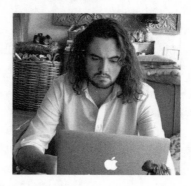

Josh: Early on in the writing process for *The Boy Between*. Little did I know that writing would have a such a positive effect on my mental health.

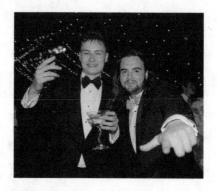

Josh: My mate Alex and I – Alex who rushed me to A&E when my wrist was cut. This is me on the other side of depression, happy to socialise and looking forward to whatever the future brings . . . I am pointing at *you* in this picture and I want to say that whatever you are going through, you've got this!

ACKNOWLEDGMENTS

The Boy Between would not have been possible were it not for the vision, support and encouragement of so many wonderful people willing to advance the difficult discussion on depression and suicide to try and help change the narrative.

Special thanks to the team at Little A and Amazon Publishing, particularly our editors, Victoria 'Pepe' Pepe-Whiting and Tiffany 'Teaseblossom' Martin, whose brutal, fearless editing helped whip this work into shape! And the wider team: Dominic, Eoin, Laura, Sana, Bekah, Hatty and everyone we have worked with – you know who you are. Thank you for taking the leap of faith! We love being part of the Little A, Amazon Family – a family not afraid to tackle the tough stuff over a cuppa and to give a voice where it is most needed. www.apub.com

Our brilliant agent, Caroline Michel at PFD, who saw the potential in our story and said, 'This is a book!' – thank you, as ever, Caroline Xx www.pfd.co.uk

The team at ED.PR for all their public relations mastery – #yourock #edpr www.edpr.co.uk

Author shots and additional photography by the very talented Paul Smith www.paulwardsmith.com

Our family – thank you all for giving us permission and support to explore such a tough subject that has touched us all, and for allowing us to pick at old wounds. I know it's been painful at times and yet your openness and dedication to help us tell this story has been invaluable. We love you all Xx

Josh's wonderful friends, including Alex, Olly, Olly and Olly, James, Jasper, Charlie Bravo, Rob, Louis, Ben and Tom – your friendship made the difference at times when it was needed the most. Thank you.

A big thank you to Audible – not only for helping bring this work to life, but also for being Josh's saviour in the darkness when all he was able to do was sit and listen to voices telling stories. The wealth of material available meant he was never alone, something for which we are both entirely grateful. www.audible.com

Dr P – the wonderful Dr P! The teacher who many years ago gave Josh a reason to walk tall. I don't think you will ever know quite what you did for Josh or for us as a family. Dr P, from the bottom of our hearts – thank you. X

Hannah Banana-GOAT – keep being you. Keep being great, I can't wait to see your brilliant future unfold. X

Mike and Em – sending love and thanks for always, Josh X

https://www.thecalmzone.net/ – Campaign Against Living Miserably – full of fantastic resources for those suffering from depression and those who care for them.

And I would just like to say to Josh's friends – you are my angels, my heroes, and I love each and every one of you more than I can say. I don't think you know what you did, but you helped save Josh's life. I am and always will be one very grateful mum.

(And yes, I am once again crying . . .) X

ABOUT THE AUTHORS

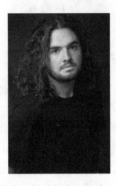

Photo © 2019 Paul Smith of Paul Smith Photography at www.paulwardsmith.com

Josiah (Josh) Hartley lives in an isolated farmhouse in the West Country, but close enough to Bristol to enjoy its music scene. He is an animal lover and servant to two French Bulldogs. Equally happy at a music festival or watching rugby with his mates, he likes the outdoor life and with Devon only a short drive away often heads to the sea to surf and sit on the beach watching the sun go down. After a stint at the University of Southampton and another at the University of Bristol and one unsuccessful suicide attempt, Josh decided to write about his descent into mental illness and the depression that has held him in its grip for the past few years. *The Boy Between* carries the overriding message that things *can* and *often do* get better. It's a book of reflection, raw, honest and full of hope: the proof being that Josh is still here and now excited about what comes next. He is ready to catch any opportunities that life throws his way, quite a thing for someone who only three years ago was living in a world gone grey, ready to disappear from the face of the earth . . .

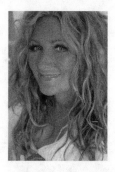

Amanda Prowse likens her own life story to those she writes about in her books. After self-publishing her debut novel *Poppy Day* in 2011, she has gone on to author twenty-five novels, six novellas and *The Boy Between*, her first work of non-fiction, co-authored with her son, Josiah Hartley. Her books have been translated into a dozen languages and she regularly tops bestseller charts all over the world. Remaining true to her ethos, Amanda writes stories of ordinary women and their families who find their strength, courage and love tested in ways they never imagined. The most prolific female contemporary fiction writer in the UK, with a legion of loyal readers, she goes from strength to strength. Being crowned 'queen of domestic drama' by the *Daily Mail* was one of her finest moments. Amanda is a regular contributor on TV and radio but her first love is, and will always be, writing. You can find her online at www.amandaprowse.com, on Twitter or Instagram @MrsAmandaProwse, and on Facebook at: www.facebook.com/AmandaProwseAuthor

ENDNOTES

1   CALM, 'Grow a Pair' (7 May 2019) Viewed 5 Jan 2020. https://www.thecalmzone.net/2019/05/seat-and-calm-grow-a-pair/

2   ITV, 'Britain Get Talking' (5 Oct 2019) Viewed 5 Jan 2020. https://www.itv.com/presscentre/press-releases/britain-get-talking-itv-announces-new-mental-wellness-campaign-help-families-get

3   MIND, 'Time to Change' Viewed 5 Jan 2020. https://www.mind.org.uk/news-campaigns/campaigns/time-to-change/

4   Mental Health America, *Mental Health Month*. Viewed 5 Jan 2020. https://www.mhanational.org/mental-health-month

5   CALM, 'CALM's view on the new ONS suicide stats' (3 Sept 2019) Viewed 5 Jan 2020. https://www.thecalmzone.net/2019/09/calms-view-on-the-new-ons-suicide-stats/

6   Matthews-King, A, 'One in eight children in England have a mental health disorder, NHS report reveals', *Independent* (22 Nov 2018) Viewed 5 Jan 2020. https://www.in-dependent.co.uk/news/health/mental-health-children-

nhs-england-depression-anxiety-report-young-people-a8646211.html

7   Science Daily, 'More than 1 in 20 US children and teens have anxiety or depression' (24 April 2018) Viewed 5 Jan 2020. https://www.sciencedaily.com/releases/2018/04/180424184119.htm

8   Ghanean H, Ceniti A K & Kennedy S H, 'Fatigue in Patients with Major Depressive Disorder: Prevalence, Burden and Pharmacological Approaches to Management', *CNS Drugs* (30 Jan 2018) Viewed 10 Jan 2020.
https://link.springer.com/article/10.1007/s40263-018-0490-z

9   The University Mental Health Charter. Viewed 19 Feb 2020. https://www.studentminds.org.uk/charter.html

10   BBC, 'Bristol University student "received no support" before death' (1 May 2019) Viewed 5 Jan 2020. https://www.bbc.co.uk/news/uk-england-bristol-48122130

11   Lightfoot L, 'A student's death: did her university do enough to help Natasha Abrahart', *Guardian* (22 Jan 2019) Viewed 5 Jan 2020. https://www.theguardian.com/education/2019/jan/22/student-death-did-university-do-enough-help-natasha-abrahart-bristol

12   Campbell D, 'Delays in NHS mental health treatment "ruining lives"', *Guardian* (9 Oct 2018. Viewed 5 Jan 2020. https://www.theguardian.com/society/2018/oct/09/mental-health-patients-waiting-nhs-treatment-delays

13 The Priory Group, 2019, 'How can Christmas affect your mental health?' Viewed 5 Jan 2020. https://www.priorygroup.com/blog/how-can-christmas-affect-your-mental-health

14 Duncan P & Davis N, 'Four million people in England are long-term users of antidepressants', *Guardian* (10 Aug 2018) Viewed 5 Jan 2020. https://www.theguardian.com/society/2018/aug/10/four-million-people-in-england-are-long-term-users-of-antidepressants

15 Sifferlin A, '13% of Americans Take Antidepressants', *Time* (15 Aug 2017) Viewed 5 Jan 2020. https://time.com/4900248/antidepressants-depression-more-common/

16 BBC, 'Bristol University students tell of mental health experiences' (29 Oct 2018) Viewed 5 Jan 2020. https://www.bbc.co.uk/news/uk-england-bristol-45976340

17 Morris S, 'Neglect by mental health trust led to Bristol student's suicide', *Guardian* (16 May 2019) Viewed 5 Jan 2020. https://www.theguardian.com/education/2019/may/16/neglect-by-mental-health-trust-led-to-bristol-students-suicide

18 College Degree Search, 'Crisis on Campus' Viewed 5 Jan 2020. http://www.collegedegreesearch.net/student-suicides/

19 The Grange Academy, 'World Mental Health Day' Viewed 5 Jan 2020. https://www.thegrangeacademy.co.uk/about_us/school_news/wordmentalhealthday/

20 Mind.org, 'Charity reveals "shocking" spend of less than 1 per cent on public mental health' (8 Dec 2016) Viewed 19 Feb

2020. https://www.mind.org.uk/news-campaigns/news/charity-reveals-shocking-spend-of-less-than-1-per-cent-on-public-mental-health/

21 Brenner E, 'The Crisis of Youth Mental Health', *Stanford Social and Innovation Review* (Spring 2019) Viewed 5 Jan 2020. https://ssir.org/articles/entry/the_crisis_of_youth_mental_health#
Note: This is for the percentage of spending on children's mental health care in the USA. Figures are difficult to determine however the *Stanford Social Innovation Review* provides useful statistics that suggest while it is better funded than the UK, the total falls woefully short of what is actually required.

22 ONS, 'Suicides in the UK: 2018 registrations' Viewed 5 Jan 2020. https://www.ons.gov.uk/peoplepopulationandcommunity/birthsdeathsandmarriages/deaths/bulletins/suicidesintheunitedkingdom/2018registrations

23 Mental Health UK, 'Suicide – Thousands of people in the UK end their lives by suicide each year' (11 Sept 2019) Viewed 5 Jan 2020. https://www.mentalhealth.org.uk/a-to-z/s/suicide

24 Samaritans.org

25 https://www.mentalhealthatwork.org.uk/

26 Villegas, L, 'How to cope with feeling stressed and overwhelmed at uni', *The Student Newspaper* (15 Nov 2017) Viewed 5 Jan 2020. https://studentnewspaper.org/how-to-cope-with-feeling-stressed-and-overwhelmed-at-uni/

27 Page L et al, 'You are not alone: student stories of mental health', *Guardian* (4 April 2014) Viewed 5 Jan 2020. https://www.theguardian.com/education/2014/apr/04/students-share-stories-of-mental-health-universities

28 Binham, C, 'UK reviews impact of student debt on financial stability' *Financial Times* (16 Jan 2019) Viewed 5 Jan 2020. https://www.ft.com/content/b189980a-19a5-11e9-9e64-d150b3105d21

29 HESA, 'Destinations of Leavers from Higher Education 2016/17' (19 July 2018) Viewed 5 Jan 2020. https://www.hesa.ac.uk/news/19-07-2018/DLHE-publication-201617

30 Hess A, 'College grads expect to earn $60,000 in their first job—here's how much they actually make', CNBC (17 Feb 2019) Viewed 20 Jan 2020. https://www.cnbc.com/2019/02/15/college-grads-expect-to-earn-60000-in-their-first-job----few-do.html

31 Friedman Z, 'Student Loan Debt Statistics In 2019: A $1.5 Trillion Crisis', *Forbes* (25 Feb 2019) Viewed 5 Jan 2020. https://www.forbes.com/sites/zackfriedman/2019/02/25/student-loan-debt-statistics-2019/#2ebb40ae133f

32 Barr S, 'Six Ways Social Media Negatively Affects Your Mental Health', *Independent* (10 Oct 2019) Viewed 5 Jan 2020. https://www.independent.co.uk/life-style/health-and-families/social-media-mental-health-negative-effects-depression-anxiety-addiction-memory-a8307196.html

33 Stubley P, 'Chemistry student dies suddenly in 13th suspected suicide at Bristol University in three years', *Independent* (10 Aug 2019) Viewed 5 Jan 2020. https://www.independent. co.uk/news/uk/home-news/student-death-suicide-bristol-university-maria-stancliffe-cook-a9051606.html

34 BBC 'Bristol students protest at mental health "crisis"' (21 Nov 2018) Viewed 5 Jan 2020. https://www.bbc.co.uk/news/ uk-england-bristol-46293109